FOCUS ON DANCE XI

Dance for the OLDER ADULT

Rayma K. Beal
Sherrill Berryman-Miller
Editors

A Project of the
National Dance Association

An Association of the
American Alliance for Health, Physical Education, Recreation, and Dance

On the cover: The Dance Exchange's "Dancers of the Third Age," directed by Liz Lerman. Photo courtesy of Bernd Uhlig, Hamburg, West Germany.

The American Alliance for Health, Physical Education, Recreation, and Dance
1900 Association Drive
Reston, Virginia 22091

ISBN 0-88314-385-2

Purposes of the American Alliance for Health, Physical Education, Recreation, and Dance

The American Alliance is an educational organization, structured for the purposes of supporting, encouraging, and providing assistance to member groups and their personnel throughout the nation as they seek to initiate, develop, and conduct programs in health, leisure, and movement-related activities for the enrichment of human life.

Alliance objectives include:

1. Professional growth and development -- to support, encourage, and provide guidance in the development and conduct of programs in health, leisure, and movement-related activities which are based on the needs, interests, and inherent capacities of the individual in today's society.

2. Communication -- to facilitate public and professional understanding and appreciation of the importance and value of health, leisure, and movement-related activities as they contribute toward human well-being.

3. Research -- to encourage and facilitate research which will enrich the depth and scope of health, leisure, and movement-related activities; and to disseminate the findings to the profession and other interested and concerned publics.

4. Standards and guidelines -- to further the continuous development and evaluation of standards within the profession for personnel and programs in health, leisure, and movement-related activities.

5. Public affairs -- to coordinate and administer a planned program of professional, public, and governmental relations that will improve education in areas of health, leisure, and movement-related activities.

6. To conduct such other activities as shall be approved by the Board of Governors and the Alliance Assembly, provided that the Alliance shall not engage in any activity which would be inconsistent with the status of an educational and charitable organization as defined in Section 501(c) (3) of the Internal Revenue Code of 1954 or any successor provision thereto, and none of the said purposes shall at any time be deemed or construed to be purposes other than the public benefit purposes and objectives consistent with such educational and charitable status.

Bylaws, Article III

Contents

II. PROGRAM MODELS

III. RESEARCH

IV. CURRICULAR PROGRAM MODELS

V. INTERGENERATIONAL DANCE

VI. RESOURCES

Contributors

Douglas Adams is Associate Professor of Christianity and the Arts at the Pacific School of Religion, Berkeley, California. *Sheila Barnett* is Director of The Jamaica School of Dance in Kingston, Jamaica. *Gwyn Barker* is a fifth grade teacher at Mt. View Elementary School, Omaha, Nebraska. *Rayma K. Beal* is Assistant Professor of Dance at the University of Kentucky, Lexington, Kentucky. *Sherrill Berryman-Miller* is Assistant Professor of Dance at Howard University, in Washington, D.C. *Jeff Bliss* is a member of Liz Lerman's Dance Exchange and Director of Community Classes. *David E. Corbin* is Associate Professor, University of Nebraska, Omaha, Nebraska. *Linda M. Deutch* is Director of First Step, a community-based rehabilitation program for people with psychiatric problems, in New London, Connecticut. *Cynthia P. Ensign* is an Assistant Professor at the University of Northern Iowa, Cedar Falls, Iowa. *Roger E. Foltz* is an Associate Professor and Chair of Music in the Department of Music at the University of Nebraska at Omaha, Omaha, Nebraska. *Leah Harpaz* is a faculty member of the Dance Department, 92nd Street YM-YWHA, in New York City and Adjunct Instructor, Baruch College in New York City. *Bernadette Hecox* is an Associate Professor in the Clinical Physical Therapy Program in Physical Therapy, Columbia University, New York, New York. *Graham Hempel* is Associate Professor of Dance at San Diego State University, in San Diego, California. *Rosebel Koss* is Past Chair, ARAPCS and Professor Emeritus, Physical Education and Recreation Department, Ramapo College, Mahwah, New Jersey. *Liz Lerman* is Director of Dance Exchange and The Dancers of the Third Age and author of *Teaching Modern Dance To Senior Citizens.* *Pamala J. Lewis* is a part-time faculty member in Dance at Connecticut College and Dance Artist for Creative Connections Mothers in Prison Program in New London, Connecticut. *Erna Caplow-Lindner* is Professor in the Department of Health, Education and Recreation, Nassau Community College and Adjunct Professor at Adelphi University in Garden City, New York. *Richard Lopez* is Associate Professor in the Department of Subject Specialization at Florida International University in Miami, Florida. *Marianne McAdam* is Project Director, Biogerentology Laboratory, Department of Preventive Medicine, University of Wisconsin, Madison, Wisconsin. *Josie Metal-Corbin* is Associate Professor, University of Nebraska, Omaha, Nebraska. *Everett Smith* is Director, Biogerentology Laboratory, Department of Preventive Medicine, University of Wisconsin, Madison, Wisconsin. *Sally K. Zook* is a graduate student, Department of Curriculum and Instruction Health Education, and a project assistant in preventive medicine in the Biogerentology Laboratory, University of Wisconsin.

Preface

Dance for the older adult is a relatively new focus of dance activity. It is new in the sense there is not an established body of knowledge for dancers working in this field. In order to address the movement needs of older adults in a creative, meaningful manner, we have gathered information from various dance styles and technical backgrounds, as well as from the fields of gerontology, physiology of exercise, psychology, and sociology.

As dancers, we have intuitively known that our active creative movements help us remain flexible and in turn help us age gracefully. Research on dance activities with older adults is beginning to confirm this hypothesis. Dance can provide physical, social, and emotional benefits to all participants no matter what their age. This book is intended to be a resource guide for individuals who are working or would like to work with older adults, regardless of dance background or training.

Dance activities can make a positive contribution to older adult activities because through dance, joints are lubricated, muscles are stretched and strengthened, and through exertion gain a release of tension and an increase in relaxation. In addition, musical selections for dance activities can be stimulating and trigger positive memories for participants. Dance activities provide social interaction in a supportive group setting. Laughter and smiles are a natural part of dance classes.

At this time we would like to acknowledge all the participants in our dance classes that have taught us how to keep our perspective on life, and what it means to be an active adult who happens to be older. We have learned as much from them as we hope they have from us.

Margie R. Hanson, Executive Director for NDA, deserves praise for initiating this project and is the model of perseverance for waiting five years to see this work completed. We also wish to thank Martin Connor, Acquisitions Editor for AAHPERD who has been instrumental and encouraging in seeing this project through; Lisa Barr, the wordprocessor for this project, whose commitment and efficiency helped to meet the publication deadline; Sandra Minton, former Publications Director for NDA, who served as an advisor to this project. Diane Milhan served as first editor, Sherrill Berryman-Miller and Josie Metal-Corbin as co-editors. When Josie went on sabbatical, Rayma K. Beal became co-editor with Sherrill. In this capacity, we accept responsibility for the contents and purposes of this book along with its possible errors. We hope you will use this resource guide to begin work or continue working with a very rewarding group of students - adults aged 60+.

Rayma K. Beal
Co-Editor

Introduction

The number of older people in the world is growing faster then the general population, and 23 nations now have more than 2 million elderly each, according to the U.S. Census Bureau. Currently 10% of our population is 65 years or older. Most of them live independently, but the quality of their living is greatly restricted by low income, poor housing, poor nutrition, and poor health which critically affect their freedom, individuality, usefulness, and independence.

When the aged become consciously aware of physical and mental deterioration, increasing dependence and debility, they unconsciously regress psychologically. Older people need incentives to restructure their lives. They need opportunities to participate with peers in meaningful activities that are validated by society.

The whole spectrum of movement is diminished for the aged. Within our system we have subtle culturally determined reinforcers which encourage negative self-images and attitudes as people grow old. Our society frequently prescribes, along with what we eat, wear, and think, even how and when we shall grow old. Individuals are often forced to assume the characteristics physical and mental attitudes of the aged, once they have acquired a certain number of years. While the Older American Act of 1965 sets the national tone of concern for the elderly by appropriating federal funds for a limited range of social services, it is the programs, research, activities, and resources that actually provide the services and opportunities for assisting this population with life and societal changes.

Focus XI is a collection of articles designed to expand the information network, identify current programs, and provide research in the field of dance/movement and gerontology. Different approaches, techniques, and philosophies are documented by individuals who are active in the field. The nation's aging population is facing their senior years with an increased awareness of the need for physical and mental activity maintenance. This document is meant to serve as a resource of the evidence that continues to mount on the positive relationship between the physical activity of dance and healthy mental attitudes. We hope that it will generate future discussion and ideas in the field.

Sherrill Berryman-Miller
Co-Editor

I. Guidelines for Activities With Older Adults

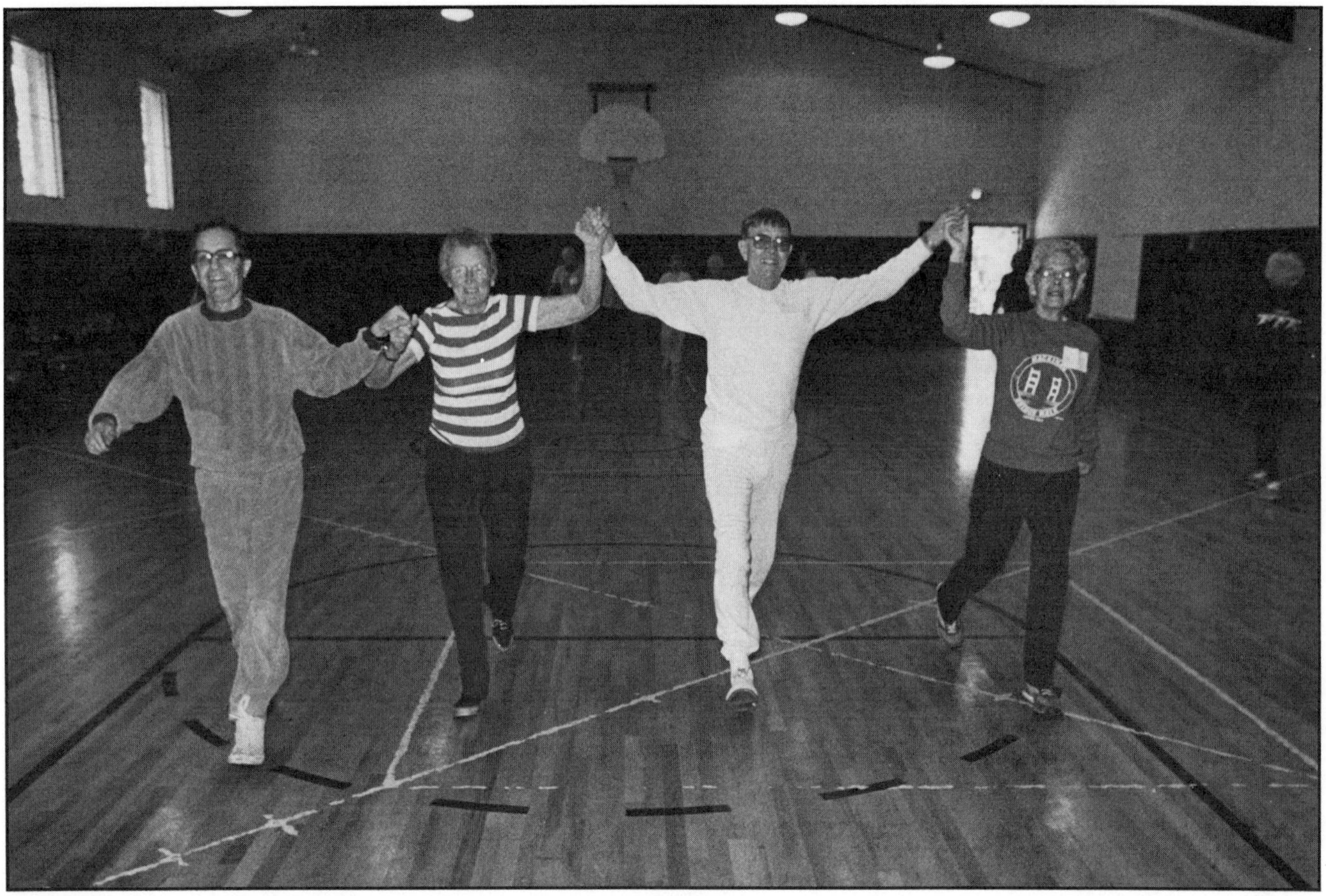

PHOTO COURTESY OF MARIANNE McADAM

To move is to be alive!

1

Moving Into The Third Age

AAHPERD Serves A New Clientele

Rosabel Koss

American society is aging. The future of our country will be shaped by trends and projections charted by the demographers (Committee on Aging, 1984). The United States is not alone in its destiny. The entire world population is growing older, presenting a challenge to education and social policy in every country. Drastic demographic changes in European societies occurred 15 to 30 years ago, while the developing countries are just now beginning to chart their older populations in the United Nations reported statistics. According to a United Nations report (1975), the number of persons in the world who are 60 or older will double during the 35-year span between 1970 and 2005.

The Abkhasians in Georgia of the Soviet Union refer to their older citizens as "Longer-Living." In Sweden, they are called, "The Pensioners." German research writes about sports, games, and exercise after forty for the "Older People." In Australia, it is "Aged Care." In China, it is "Elder Care" and everyone, including the elderly, seems to have a particular job to do that is necessary for the good of the entire society (Missinni, 1983). Longevity rates vary among the nations and appear to be the result of heredity and lifestyles (Elrick, 1978).

The elderly in the United States have grown from approximately 3,000,000 in 1965 [four percent of the population] to 25,000,000 in 1980, more than 11 percent of the population. The fastest growing segment of the older population is 74 years and older, many of whom are women. This shift in age composition has resulted in burgeoning health care delivery costs and growing public awareness of the potential problems, and realities of aging. There is widespread interest and concern about the quality of life for older Americans.

Demographers forecast an uneven rate of change for the over-65 population. Americans will enjoy a period for the next 30 years when there will be sustained but undramatic growth. But beginning in 2010, the aging of the "baby boom" generation, an older society will suddenly be with us, whether we are prepared for it nor not! If we want things better for ourselves and our children, now is the time for unified action--not optimistic and pious rhetoric, but a fully researched and carefully stated policy that reflects the desires of the total citizenry and allows for the implementation of more effective programs to meet the needs of older people.

A new focus

Early AAHPERD services focused on college and university youth. Later we discovered the need to work with high school students, and only then did it become obvious that early childhood was most important. The increasing interest in programs for older citizens became evident when a presidential Committee On Aging was appointed in 1974. The task was to develop a knowledge base and formulate a process for sensitizing AAHPERD to our own aging, motivating our professional colleagues to serve a new clientele in our communities and developing model programs in colleges and universities throughout the nation.

We were being asked to serve a new clientele by stretching our resources and creativity to develop community programs based in schools, colleges, and universities. At the same time we must increase the number and quality of programs nationwide which prepare students for careers in health, fitness, and leisure for an aging population. AAHPERD must serve as a clearinghouse for research, consultation, and dissemination of information concerning health and fitness for the older population.

By 1985 the task was well under way. The latest Directory (1984) shows 196 programs in 46 states and the District of Columbia. The Alliance Board of Governors voted in April 1985 to provide a new structure for those members working with the aging population. The Council On Aging and Adult Development has become a part of The Association For Research, Administration, Professional Councils, and Societies (ARAPCS).

To move is to be alive!

Over the years health educators, physical educators, coaches, dancers and choreographers, therapists, and leisure and recreation specialists have proposed many purposes for human movement (Westen, 1962). Such natural movements as walking, running, and jumping were first defined by Guts Muth (Germany 1759-1830). This so-called natural system was further developed in Denmark and Great Britain. In Sweden, Per Hendrik Ling (1776-1833) gave movement an anatomical direction when he developed medical gymnastics, for sick and well people, which required exercising all muscles and joints in a set order. Neils Bukh (Denmark 1880-1950) saw the aim "to regain and maintain man's natural suppleness, strength, and agility, so that these powers may have an opportunity of developing bodily beauty, harmony, and effective purposeful action. Skeletal stiffness should give way to mobility, weakness of musculature to strength, and awkwardness to agility" (Westen, 1962).

Muska Mosston (1965) described three categories of values. The *assigned value* belongs to the dancers and choreographers who attribute a feeling, an idea, or a mood to a movement. *Functional value* is the domain of the coach or sport enthusiast where specific movements are required for particular skills. The *intrinsic value* of movement is concerned with the intentional development of physical attributes or components required to develop and maintain a healthy mind and body. It would appear, for the elderly, that all three goals would be appropriate, but a necessity for successful aging is an understanding of the separate components of total fitness, especially the intrinsic value because it is often the difference between remaining independent or becoming dependent.

Ideally, preparation for a physically fit old age should being in youth in order to accrue maximum benefits. Exercise is not necessarily to prolong life but rather to increase the years of feeling good.

De Vries (1975) concludes that "all of the important factors that lead to good health are under our control. We must accept the responsibility."

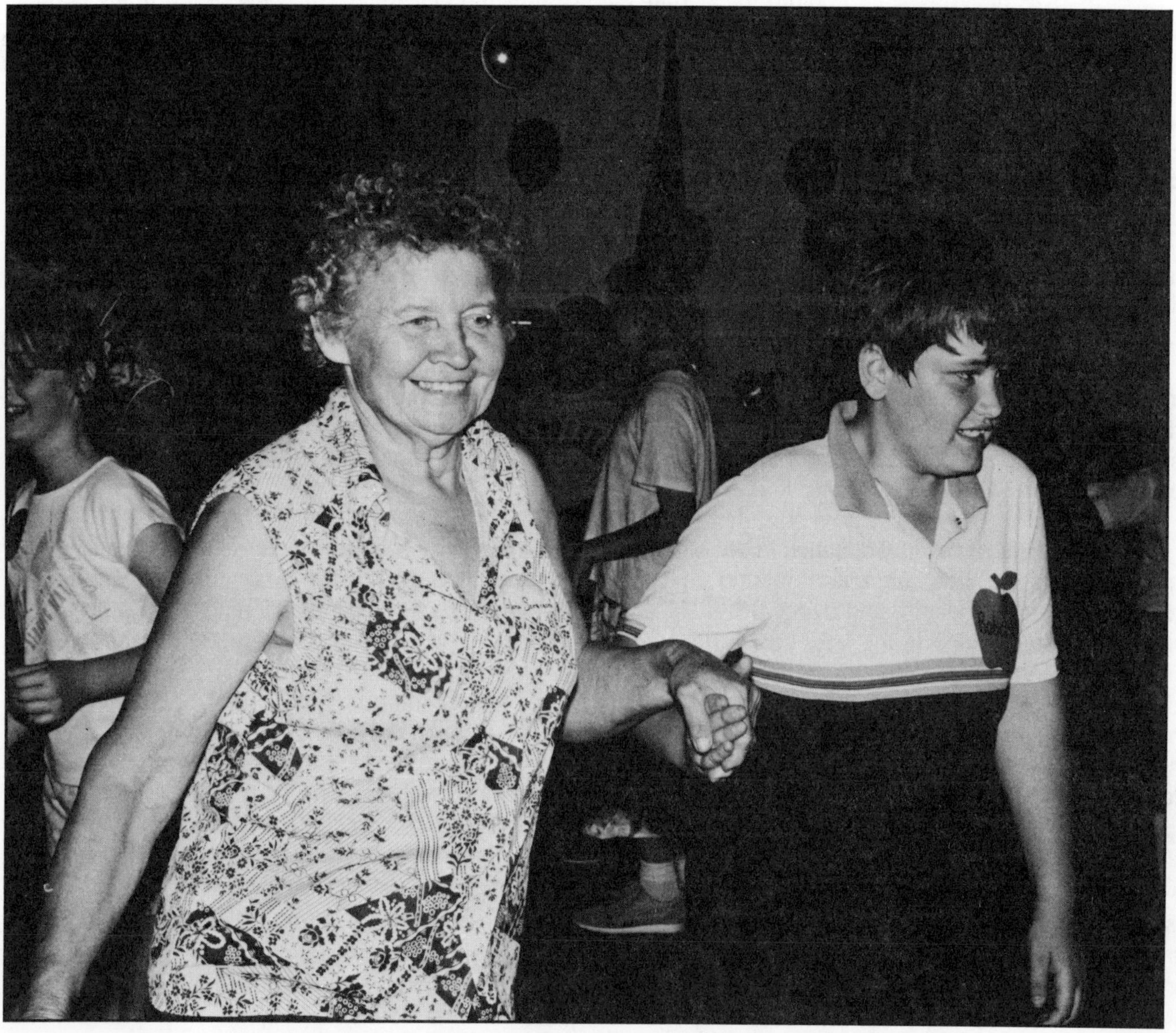

PHOTO COURTESY OF DAVID E. CORBIN

Older adults are a valuable resource of ethnic and historical material that can be passed on, through dance, to younger generations.

In 1976 de Vries stated before the Senate Sub-Committee On Aging, "In view of the many benefits likely to result from the improvement of physical fitness in the elderly, it seems desirable to begin the implementation of programs of exercise, nutrition, and stress reduction or relaxation procedures. However, training of older people in these areas requires instructors with highly specialized preparation and skills. At the present time, it is this resource that is lacking."

Professionals need to get involved

Since the de Vries testimony in 1976, AAHPERD members have been at work developing professional preparation programs and materials. Research and sports medicine has moved forward. Corrective therapy and laboratories to study the physiology of exercise have been developed.

There is every indication that seniors of the future will require and demand trained leadership in health and exercise as a form of preventive medicine. Model programs for older citizens can be arranged to fit the needs of the least able, sitting in chairs; the more able, moving around a strong base of support; and the most able who can move freely through space. Professionals of the future must be prepared to provide the necessary leadership.

Teachers of health education in the elementary and secondary schools would do well to involve their students in multigenerational learning experiences, to emphasize the life-cycle concept, and to add units on aging, death, and dying. Physical educators can concentrate on developing lifelong skills for health and satisfaction in the later years. In American colleges and universities the most recent course offerings are in aging, death, dying, fitness, and the physiology of exercise. Gerontology specialties are developing. On the community level, continuing education, senior centers, adult day care centers and nursing homes need leadership. Elderhostel or some sort of vacation college for older students, counseling for career changes, and preretirement seminars are in vogue. All offer creative leadership roles for AAHPERD professionals of the future. We need to become involved.

The National Health Promotion Initiative, sponsored jointly by a memorandum between the United States Public Health Service and the Administration On Aging, will motivate seniors and those who hire the care-givers to search for leadership in the areas of exercise, nutrition, drug and substance abuse, and accident prevention. These priorities have been set at the national level. AAHPERD is involved in the Health Promotion Initiative as a member of The National Volunteer Organization for the Independent Living of the Aging (NVOILA), sponsored by the National Council On Aging.

The challenge is one we cannot fail to meet. The aged are sensitive barometers of how well a society handles the basic problems of living. Polarization of the generations must be avoided, new specialties developed, and greater understanding and sensitivity need to grow among the young so that the aging population can utilize education for the necessary adaptation to new lifestyles, and better health.

REFERENCES

de Vries, H. A. (1975). Physiology of Exercise and Aging. In Woodrull and Berren, *Concepts and Issues In Gerontology* (Chapter 12). New York: Van Nostrand.

de Vries, H. A. (1976, March). Testimony Before Senate Sub-committee On Aging. p. 718 (Report No. 55-648, 0-75-46).

Elrick, H. et al. (1978). *Living Longer and Better.* Mountain View, CA: World Publications.

Missinni, L. (1983). Aging In China. *Perspectives On Aging.* National Council On Aging, 11(6).

Mosston, M. (1965). *Development Movement.* Columbus, OH: Charles E. Merrill.

Price & O (1984). *A National Directory of Physical Fitness Programs For Older Adults* (2nd ed.) Saranac Lake, NY: North Country Community College Press.

United Nations (1975). *The Aging: Trends and Policies.* New York: United Nations Department of Economics and Social Affairs.

United States Senate Special Committee On Aging in conjunction with American Association of Retired Persons (1984). *Aging In America. Trends and Projections.* Washington, DC: U.S. Government Printing Office.

Westen, A. (1962). *The Making of American Physical Education.* New York: Appleton-Century.

2

An Overview Of Dance

Cynthia P. Ensign

As a brief introduction to the history of modern dance, I often tell my students that dance has come full circle. People first danced to express themselves, to move simply for the joy of movement, and often to feel a sense of community with others. Today, people can express their humanness through modern dance --a medium available to men and women of all shapes, sizes, and ages. But modern dance is only one of the many dance forms which offer these benefits.

Some possible choices of dance forms would include folk, square, ballroom, ballet, modern, jazz, tap, soft-shoe, aerobic, country-western, and clogging. Because of the high-level technical skill traditionally required in some forms, the demand for them may be less. Seniors, however, may still gain some benefits from those forms.

Through ballet, for instance, seniors may improve their posture and decrease their lower back pain. They may also improve their coordination and gain a sense of accomplishment from being able to put together a series of steps in a ballet combination. And who isn't captivated by the rhythms of Bill "Bojangles" Robinson? Although a senior may never become a Bojangles or a Fred Astaire, the experience of working with rhythms can be exciting and challenging.

Men and women of all ages

The classification senior, senior adult, senior citizen, the elderly, and the aging can encompass a large age span. Usually the classification includes those 55 and older, but that can mean including those from 55 to 100 -- a range of 45 years. Imagine placing newborns and 45-year-olds, or 20 to 65-year-olds, in the same classification. Lumping seniors in a single category without further considerations can be limiting and contrary to their abilities and needs.

Level of ability does not necessarily correspond to age. A young senior who is just beginning to become active in movement may be mixed in a group with a much older person who has been active throughout a lifetime. Programs, therefore, need to be designed which recognize the different physical, psychological, and social needs of the many individuals who fall within the broad classification of senior. In many instances, the physical demands of an activity can be adapted so that all participants can benefit at their own levels.

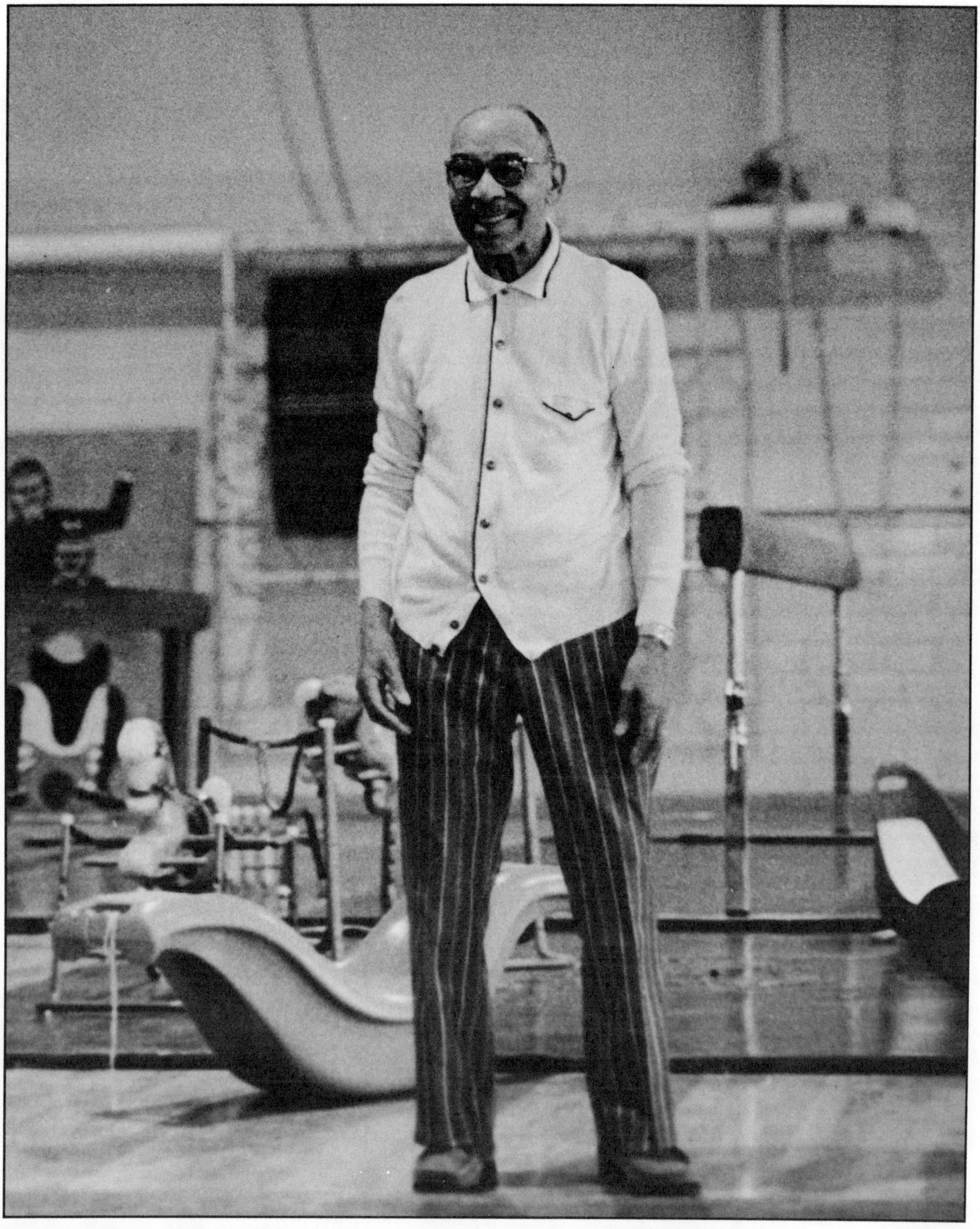

Participation in dance can renew self-esteem and provide the older adult with a sense of achievement.

Physical benefits

Because of the uniqueness of dance and because of the present emphasis on fitness, several physical benefits have been documented. They include improvement in flexibility, muscle strength and endurance, cardiovascular endurance, balance, coordination, and agility. Increased bone mineral content and kinesthetic awareness have been noted, as well as decreased difficulty with arthritis, insomnia, neuromuscular hypertension, stress-related diseases, and low back pain. Weight and diabetes are more easily controlled when individuals are physically active (Corbin and Metal-Corbin, 1983; Smith and Gilligan, 1983; Stenger and Smith, 1985).

Psychological benefits

Much research is being conducted in sports psychology. Many of the benefits found in these studies will probably apply to all age groups, including the senior adult. Some of the psychological benefits gained from participation in dance are increased self-confidence, self-esteem, stability, sense of achievement, acceptance by others, expression of feelings, recognition of creative abilities, and decreased depression (Corbin and Metal-Corbin, 1983; Stenger and Smith, 1985).

Social benefits

Senior adults may find themselves increasingly alone. Retirement often eliminates daily personal contacts with others; spouses and close friends may die; and today's mobile society may mean that children and grandchildren no longer live in the immediate vicinity. For the senior, having the opportunity to be with peers can be very rewarding. Social benefits gained from participating in dance classes include decreased isolation, loneliness, and boredom; and increased sharing, support, tactile contact, cooperation, and fun (Corbin and Metal-Corbin, 1983; Stenger and Smith, 1985).

REFERENCES

Corbin, D.E., & Metal-Corbin, J. (1983). *Reach for it! A handbook of exercise and dance activities for older adults.* Dubuque, Iowa: Eddie Bowers Publishing Co.

Smith, E., & Gilligan, C. (1983, August). Physical activity prescription for the older adult. *The Physician and Sportsmedicine*, 11, 91-101.

Stenger, L., & Smith, C.M. (1985). *Healthy moves for older adults.* Washington, DC: ERIC Clearinghouse on Teacher Education.

3

Guidelines for Using Dance with Older Adults

Richard Lopez

Older adults, in particular, benefit from regular exercise because regular exercise retards deterioration of fitness that occurs with aging and inactivity (Serfass, 1981). Dance is a good exercise for a well-balanced exercise program for older adults. In addition to its commonalities with other aerobic activities, dance has several unique advantages. Dance can be conducted with little equipment in a limited facility. It poses few health risks. Vigorous arm movements can be combined with leg movements. Exercising the arm and shoulder muscles as well while frequently changing locomotor patterns and movement direction also provides a full, even use of leg muscles. Such variations also reduce the repetitive stress placed on any single area of the limb and thereby decreases the possibility of overstress injuries (Pruett & Lopez, 1982).

While participation in a well-designed program can be beneficial, participation in a poor one is dangerous. Exercise of an inappropriate type, duration, intensity, frequency, and progression can trigger a cardiovascular accident or serious musculoskeletal injury (ACSM, 1980). It is the dance/exercise leader's responsibility to prescribe and supervise a program which minimizes danger. To assist leaders, the American Alliance Committee on Aging has established guidelines for leaders of exercise programs for older adults (See Chapter 4). Dance as a primary focus for a exercise program for older adults can readily be adapted to meet the guidelines of the Alliance's Committee on Aging.

The first guideline suggests that participants complete a medical examination prior to beginning an exercise program. Ideally a physician knowledgeable in exercise physiology and the values and risks of regular exercise for older adults should conduct the examination. For programs involving vigorous exercises which exceed the intensity of everyday activities, the examination should assess the participant's ability to exercise with minimal risk to the cardiovascular, respiratory and musculoskeletal systems. A physician can assess physiological response to exercise through an exercise test--such as a functional graded exercise test--which monitors the cardiovascular response (heart rate, EKG, and blood pressure) to progressively increasing intensities of exercise. In addition, the American College of Sports Medicine recommends that the screening exam include personal and surgical history, assessment of cardiovascular risk factors, resting electocardiogram, resting systolic and diastolic pressure, blood counts and lipid analysis. Participants should have their personal physician's approval for programs involving low level activity which does not exceed the intensity of everyday activities.

The second Committee on Aging guideline is that the type, intensity, duration, frequency, and progression of exercise be prescribed according to each participant's physiological capacity. The type of exercise is selected according to the individual's functional physical activity, interests, availability of time, equipment, and facilities.

A balanced exercise program should include aerobic activities for cardiovascular development and fat loss, stretching exercises for flexibility, and calisthentic or resistance exercises of the upper and lower body for muscular endurance and strength. Fitness level determines the rate or intensity of work. The intensity of exercise which is monitored, using the exercise heart rate as the guideline, is usually set at 60 to 90% of the maximum heart rate. The duration of the aerobic activity, which depends on the intensity, is generally between 15 to 60 minutes. The aerobic activity is followed by a 5 to 10 minute cool down.

The frequency of conditioning is generally three to five days per week. When initiating an exercise program, it is best to begin with three alternate days a week, to minimize muscle, bone, and joint discomfort. The rate of progression (the rate of increasing total work per session) depends on the stress of exercise.[3] Normally, the most rapid conditioning effects occur during the first six to eight weeks of the exercise program. During this time the total work done per session is increased approximately 5 to 10% every one to two weeks. After the rapid initial improvement, the work load is increased every two or three weeks until a caloric expenditure of 300 Kcal per session is reached (400 Kcal/session if weight loss is a primary goal). Note that adaptation to conditioning takes approximately 40% longer or an additional week to adapt to a new work load for each decade in life after age 30.

Dance is a good exercise mode for an older adults' program because individuals can limit range of motion activities and pacing as the second guideline suggests. By restricting the range of motion, participants work within the functional limits of their joints, minimizing joint discomfort and injury while improving flexibility. During breaks between musical pieces or sections of the class, participants may monitor their heart rates, check for symptoms of fatigue, and enjoy a short rest. The dance leader can also observe participants for signs of fatigue. Thus in a dance session, an interval approach which alternates intervals of work with intervals of rest and gradually increases the amount of exercise may be employed. An interval approach permits participants to complete more work at the desired intensity.

Because the intensity of exercise is prescribed in terms of an exercise heart rate and the rate of exercise progression is adjusted according to the exercise heart rate, participants should learn to monitor their own heart rates by palpitation. Given the prescribed exercise or target rate each participant adjusts exercise intensity accordingly. Participants monitor their heart rates periodically and if necessary notify the exercise leader of any unusual responses including a failure to lower the heart rate following a lowering of the rate of work. To minimize the risk of cardiovascular or musculoskeletal injury, it is advisable to increase the work load primarily by increasing the *duration* of the work rather than the intensity. Because of the flexibility of their materials, dance leaders can easily increase work load duration without the increasing intensity.

Unlike endurance sports, dance can easily include the three components of a training session recommended by the American College of Sports Medicine: warm-up, an endurance activity, and a cool down. The warm-up includes joint readiness exercises and low level aerobic activities. Slow controlled dance movements which require a full range of motion at the joints prepare the muscles and joints by stretching the muscles and connective tissue. Dance examples may include Limon-type swings for neck and spine, head rolls, and forward and side bending of the upper and lower extremities. Low intensity aerobic movements can increase muscle and connective tissue temperature making them more pliable, gradually preparing the cardiovascular system for more intense aerobic activities. Examples include selected folk dances, especially kolos and line dances of various types. Also by adding resistance to some of these movements, through the use of props or partners, participants can increase strength and muscular endurance as well.

The second component of the exercise session, endurance, consists of aerobic activities. If improvement of cardiovascular fitness is the goal set by the older adult participants, the movers exercise at an intensity of 60 to 90% of their maximal heart rate for 15 to 60 minutes. Low level fitness individuals work at a lower intensity for a longer duration which presents fewer cardiovascular and musculoskeletal risks.

The cool down, which concludes the exercise session, consists of activities of progressively diminishing intensity and some additional stretch work. The cool down prevents a pooling of blood in the lower extremities and stretches the muscles used during the exercise session. Both goals of the cool down are met by using slower musical pieces and incorporating slow, controlled stretching movements.

The third Alliance guideline is to have a well-defined emergency plan. Exercise leaders should be trained in cardio-pulmonary resuscitation techniques (CPR). Someone trained in CPR should be present or nearby during every exercise session, and participants should be trained to assist in an emergency.

In addition to monitoring heart rates, participants should be taught to identify signs of exertional intolerance (dizziness, angina, nausea, respiratory difficulty, and unusual fatigue or pain) and realize the need to report these signs to the exercise or dance leader. In addition to looking for these signs, the exercise or dance leader should look for any signs of staggering, facial expressions, signifying severe distress, loss of vigor, and severe pallor. The participants should know whom to contact and emergency phone numbers should be visible.

REFERENCES

Alliance Committee on Aging. Guidelines for Exercise Programs for Older Adults. Reston, VA: Author, 1981.

American College of Sports Medicine. *Guidelines for graded exercise testing and exercise prescription.* Philadelphia: Lea and Febiger, 1980.

Pruett, D. and Lopez, R. *Florida Journal of Health, Physical Education, Recreation and Dance*, August 1982, pp. 10-11.

Serfass, R.C. Exercise for the elderly: what are the benefits and how do we get started? In E.L. Smith and R.C. Serfass (Eds.) *Exercise and aging: The scientific basis.* Hillside, NJ: Enslow Publishers, 1981, pp. 121-27.

4

Guidelines For Exercise Programs For Older Persons (Age 50 And Older)

As Developed By The American Alliance For Health, Physical Education, Recreation And Dance

There can be risk in sudden, unregulated and injudicious use of exercise. However, the risk can be minimized through proper preliminary screening and individualized prescribing of exercise programs. It is important for older persons entering an exercise program to have a medical evaluation by a physician knowledgeable about physical exercise and its implications.

For programs involving vigorous exercises (i.e., exercises that exceed the level of intensity encountered in normal daily activities, such as walking and climbing stairs), the medical evaluation should insure that the individual can participate in vigorous exercise without any undue risk to the cardiovascular and other bodily systems. Normally, a test that ascertains an individual's cardiorespiratory adjustment to the stress of exercise is an advisable part of the examination. Minimally, it would ascertain if the cardiovascular system, by such appropriate indicators as heart rate and blood pressure, can adequately adjust to vigorous exercise (i.e., exercises that do not exceed the level of intensity encountered in normal daily activities), participants should have their personal physician's approval.

Regardless of whether or not a program of exercise is vigorous or of low intensity, the following guidelines to insure the safety of the participants are offered:

1. In that each person's response to the stress of exercise is specific to that individual, it is important that each person's response to exercise be monitored periodically for signs of undue stress (unduly high heart rate, nausea, dyspnea, pallor, pain). Participants should be taught to monitor their own heart rate and to recognize these indicators of stress. Unusual responses should be reported to the exercise leader immediately. Exercise leaders, also, should be vigilant of these warning signs.

2. Every exercise program must have a well-defined emergency plan for exercise leaders to follow in the event of cardiac arrest or other accidents.

3. Exercise programs must have adequate supervision. Exercise leaders should be trained in Cardiopulmonary Resuscitation (CPR) techniques. At the very minimum, CPR trained personnel should be present during every exercise session or in close proximity to the exercise program.

Approved: Alliance Committee on Aging 4-14-81, Boston, MA; Alliance Board of Governors, 10-4-81, Reston, VA.

5

Dance As A Vehicle To Fitness For The Healthy Older Adult

Marianne McAdam

Dance is known for its beauty and ability to express our thoughts in its art form, to provide joy in its social form, and psychological benefits in its creative and therapeutic form. Although we all acknowledge the physical benefits derived from dance, this has not been its purpose.

Today many fitness enthusiasts have discovered the joys and benefits of rhythmic movement and have termed it "Aerobic Dance" (Garrick et al., 1986). It has commonly been practiced by a young population, danced to rock music, and characterized by jazzy movements and an excess of hops, jumps, and jogging in place (Richie et al., 1985). Unfortunately, "Aerobic Dance" has often been taught by instructors with little or no dance or injury prevention training and with little creativity (Vetter et at., 1985). These shortcomings have caused its poor reputation among dance educators and artists who resent the fact that the word "dance" is used to describe what many would call "calisthenics to music".

Our choice as dancers is either to ignore the fitness craze and lose exposure to many people we would otherwise never see, or join in, and do it better. The older adult is an example of a population that can greatly benefit from the dancer's expertise and creativity and yet is rarely involved in our dance classes. Many danced in the Big Band days but have not danced since and find it a threatening proposition to begin again. Few have ever had the experience of creative movement and in fact many have never seen a live performance of dance in its art form.

The older adult is an ideal student for the dance educator. There is no other age group that has more to offer to dance in terms of life experience and wisdom. Retirement gives them the time to get involved in regular dance classes and endurance dance can give them what they need to maintain the quality of their lives. An exercise class can lure people normally inhibited by dance, and a good dance educator can expose them in an unthreatening manner to the joys of all forms of movement. Before long all realize that exercising in any other manner would not compare to the fun of dancing.

An added benefit to exposing new people to dance is the chance of creating a larger audience for the art of dance. This age group is incredibly appreciative of what a good teacher gives them and become extremely loyal. If their teacher is involved in a performance, they will be there showing their support and gratitude. Their new exposure to and appreciation of dance can break down (commonly held) negative, stereotypic images of who we are and what we do. Having experienced movement themselves many become "hooked" on dance and become some of our most tireless supporters.

The dancer has much to offer to a movement class focussed on improving fitness. First is a fundamental understanding of movement that few physical educators, physical therapists or any other professionals who teach exercise share. This allows the dancer to create movement specific to and appropriate for the group and the individuals within it. Their vast experience with movement offers endless possibilities from which to create interesting and varied classes. Composition skills, familiarity with music, rhythmic abilities and an understanding of how to teach movement are invaluable to offering an interesting, safe and creative exercise class.

My exposure to the area of "dance/exercise" came unexpectedly with an excellent job offer at the University of Wisconsin-Madison's Biogerontology Lab following the completion of my Masters Degree in Dance Education. For 6 years I have worked in a research study under the direction of Everett L. Smith evaluating the effects of exercise on bone density in women (age 35-70) (Smith & Raab, 1986). The challenge was to design a program that would be safe, and interesting enough to keep 110 women exercising 3x a week for 4 years. What the staff (all of whom have strong backgrounds in dance) developed is a form of creative dance exercise which we have labeled "Endurance Dance" to distinguish it clearly from the typical Aerobic Dance. The program has proven to be safe, effective, and thoroughly enjoyable for the participants. This article will describe Endurance Dance as it is used with the older adult with the necessary modifications which we have learned through our ongoing classes and research in the Biogerontology Lab with people 65 and older (Agre et al. 1987 & Raab et al. 1987).

Speaking from experience, the endurance dance class is quite a change for the ballet or modern dance teacher. Where the normal dance class would focus on technique the exercise class offers movement on a grosser level with attention to technique more often only as it relates to the prevention of injury. For example, in the "across the floor" section of a modern dance class the purpose would be to perfect the dancers performance of a particular movement. In the class, focused on fitness, the teacher could use similar movements but with the emphasis on keeping the students moving.

Although dancers are generally a very fit sector of our population, most have not had the time or opportunity to study exercise physiology and therefore do not understand why cardiovascular fitness is so critical to health. The University of Wisconsin - Madison dance major program is a good example of this dilemma. The curriculum has a strong emphasis in the sciences including Anatomy, Physiology, Kinesiology; but Exercise Physiology is not required because of the already overwhelming course load. Therefore, the remainder of this paper will present some of the basic exercise physiology and precautions the dancer will need to understand to teach the exercise oriented dance class to the older adult. Ideas for the class format, content, and curriculum will be discussed give the the dancer a start to venture into a new and different form of dance.

Endurance Exercise

Aerobics have become commonly used to denote exercises that utilize oxygen throughout the movement yet push the body to the point that it must improve to meet the new demands. Aerobics are activities such as swimming, running, brisk walking, cross country skiing, and some forms of dance. Intense, start-stop type activities like sprinting and power lifting are termed anaerobic and use a metabolic pathway that does not use oxygen and therefore cannot be continued for any length of time (McArdle et al., 1981).

The technique to making a dance class aerobic is to provide exercise with adequate intensity, frequency, and duration. Research has indicated that to improve cardiorespiratory function significantly a person must work at 65%-85% of their maximum heart rate reserve and exercise at this level 3-4 times a week for 20-30 minutes (Pollack et al., 1978).

Many older people believe that exercising in such a manner is unnatural and therefore unnecessary. However, today, when our daily lives require less and less physical activity, an "artificial" form of exercise often becomes necessary if the quality of life is to be maintained. Appropriate exercise can improve the quality of life by providing people the endurance, strength, and range of motion necessary to complete their chosen activities. A person's level of fitness can make the difference between whether he or she can climb the stairs to the bedroom or complete house, lawn, and garden chores. This, of course, can make the difference between independent and dependent living in later years (Shepard, 1978). Considering that in the U.S. population over the age of 65 is expected to grow from approximately 12% in 1987 to 15% in the year 2000, a healthy elderly population becomes important to avoid the burden of large health care costs on the entire society (Brody & Brock, 1985).

Research on aging is an exciting field today, showing that as much as 50% of the aging process may actually be caused by disuse (Smith, 1984). Research indicates that with adequate and appropriate exercise the older adult improves in aerobic capacity, strength, range of motion, neuromuscular coordination, and bone strength and density (Topics in Geriatric Rehabilitation, 1985). Bone density is a particularly important issue because of loss of bone, or Osteoporosis, causes approximately 1.3 million fractures a year for women at the cost of 3-6 million dollars (NIH, 1984). A growing number of studies are now showing that with adequate calcium and proper exercise bone loss may be retarded significantly, therefore, decreasing the risk of fracture (Smith and Gilligan, 1987).

A well-trained, enthusiastic dance instructor can provide a dance class that results in many of the above benefits and at the same time is safe, creative, and enjoyable. A sedentary group of people previously uninterested in exercise will need a form of exercise that takes their minds off of the fact that they are exercising. Dance is an effective method of distraction! Once people have experienced the benefits of exercise and understand proper technique, they are more likely to continue to make exercise and dance a part of their lives.

Safety Precautions and the Target Heart Rate

One of the first priorities when beginning an endurance dance class is to determine accurately the abilities and fitness level of your participants. The high probability of disease and disability among this age group necessitates a more careful health assessment than might be required for other age groups. Therefore, it is recommended that the teacher require a medical history from each participant and preferably, a doctor's approval (Smith and Gilligan, 1983).

The next step is to be sure your classes are organized by functional ability and not chronological age. A 70 year old who walks several miles a day and a 70 year old who barely has the strength to perform daily tasks would need very different types of movement classes. This paper focuses on the former group, although aerobic exercise and a creative, total fitness program is just as important for the chair-ridden adult. Many of the following ideas can be modified and used for such people.

Determining a heart rate level of intensity each person should work allows many individuals of varying fitness levels to exercise safely together in a class situation yet see cardiovascular improvement. This level of intensity is termed the Training Heart Rate (THR) and can be determined by the following formula (Smith and Gilligan, 1983).

THR = % LEVEL/100 X (maximum heartrate - resting heartrate) + resting heart rate

Ideally, maximum heart rate is measured by a maximum work capacity test. Otherwise, maximum heart rate may be estimated as 220 - age. (Note: this should be adjusted when drugs that lower heart rate, such as beta blockers, are used.) Resting heart rate should be taken first thing in the morning while sitting and before drinking coffee.

The intensity of the exercise as well as the duration can gradually be increased as the participant's fitness improves. The % level as noted in the formula can begin at 65 and increase for some people over a period of years to 85. Depending on the level of fitness of the participants, the duration of aerobic exercises may begin with a period of 5-10 minutes and take several months or years to increase to 20-30 minutes at their THR's.

Many people have never or rarely experienced working at this intensity and will have a difficult time continuing for even five minutes at the start of a program. Varying the level of activity within that 5-10 minute period at first will gradually allow people to adjust to working so intensely.

Increasing the intensity level of a class slowly is also important in minimizing stress to the joints. The heart and lungs are often ready for a greater intensity before the bone structure has strengthened to meet the new demand. Time is needed to strengthen the muscles surrounding the joints so they can aid in alleviating stress on them. Injury can result from a program that progresses too quickly.

Monitoring heart rates and comparing them to an individual's calculated THR will give everyone a way to monitor the intensity of a workout. Gradually participants will learn to listen to their bodies and discover what it feels like to exercise at their given THR. This allows many people at varying levels of fitness to work safely in a group situation.

Teaching older adults to take their heart rates accurately and understand the concept of training heart rate can take a great deal of time and concentrated effort. They must be taught to find either the carotid or radial pulse, whichever they find easier, counting zero for the first pulse felt and every beat thereafter for the next 10 seconds. Although difficult, they must eventually become proficient at taking a pulse while walking slowly. This assures that the heart rate measured will be as close as possible to an accurate assessment of the exercise heart rate.

A 10 second pulse is commonly used rather than a 15 second or longer pulse because the recovery period has not usually been long enough to significantly lower the pulse. The formula given determines the THR for one minute, which then needs to be divided by 6 to find the THR for 10 seconds:

10 SECOND THR = 1 MINUTE THR/6

The Endurance Dance Class

An effective endurance dance class needs to provide a total fitness program. Endurance exercise is important but strength, flexibility, balance, and coordination are also essential for fitness and injury prevention.

Ideally a class should be 50 minutes to an hour, which allows time for a 10-15 minute warm up, 10-30 minutes of aerobics, a 5 minute cool down and 10-30 minutes of strength and flexibility work. The times of each section of the class will vary with the needs and abilities of the class participants. Finishing with strength and flexibility exercises works well for the older adult. This sequence allows them to leave class relaxed and with a resting heart rate.

The class should include a number of dance styles and activities as well as a variety of music. Both the music and the dances need to be chosen according to the preferences and abilities of the participants. Ideas for movement can be drawn from all forms of dance including ballet, modern, creative, ballroom, folk, and square dance. Certain forms of dance will lend themselves better to the warmup or cooldown while others will work well for the aerobic portion of the class. International and American folk dance music is always a hit along with big band, musicals, ragtime, novelty, classical and easy listening music.

The Warmup

The warmup can be a time of creativity and constant variation from class to class. The object of this pre-aerobic time is gradually to elevate the heart rate toward the training level and to prepare the joints and muscles for the more vigorous parts of class.

Depending on the abilities of the group, the warmup can vary between classes, from moving around the room, sitting on the floor or chairs, or standing in place. Simple joint rotations and flexion/extension type exercises for each body part are a good start. Thorough stretching of the calves, hamstrings, quadriceps and back before the aerobics is also essential. Although stretching cool muscles will not as effectively increase flexibility as will stretching muscles warmed from vigorous activity, it may help prevent injury by slowly warming the muscle and increasing its range of motion to normal limits.

Using props or toys adds excitement and variety to the class. It also precipitates movement not normally performed and tends to distract people from the difficulty of exercise. Toys can include yarn balls, parachutes, Frisbees, rubber tubing, Hula Hoops, fabric (scarves), gymnastic ribbons and musical instruments (i.e. drums, tambourines, etc.). Instructors should experiment or "play" with the toys to discover movement possibilities, while keeping in mind the object of the movement is to prepare the body for the more vigorous exercise to follow. Including seemingly crazy ideas like circling the Frisbee on a finger while circling the ankle prepares the ankle for exercise. This also works on balance and coordination and begins to warm the whole body, because people are constantly stooping to pick the dropped Frisbee from the floor and beginning again.

Music for the warmup can be used as background to create a certain mood or chosen for a particular tempo or rhythm. Walking-tempo music works well for a moving warmup while quiet easy listening would work well for a floor warmup.

The warmup can also be used to teach dances or give instructions for activities that will be used in the aerobic portions of the class. The steps can be explained thoroughly and practiced slowly so they can be performed later in the class. Helping people to feel comfortable with dance steps will decrease frustration and allow for a better workout.

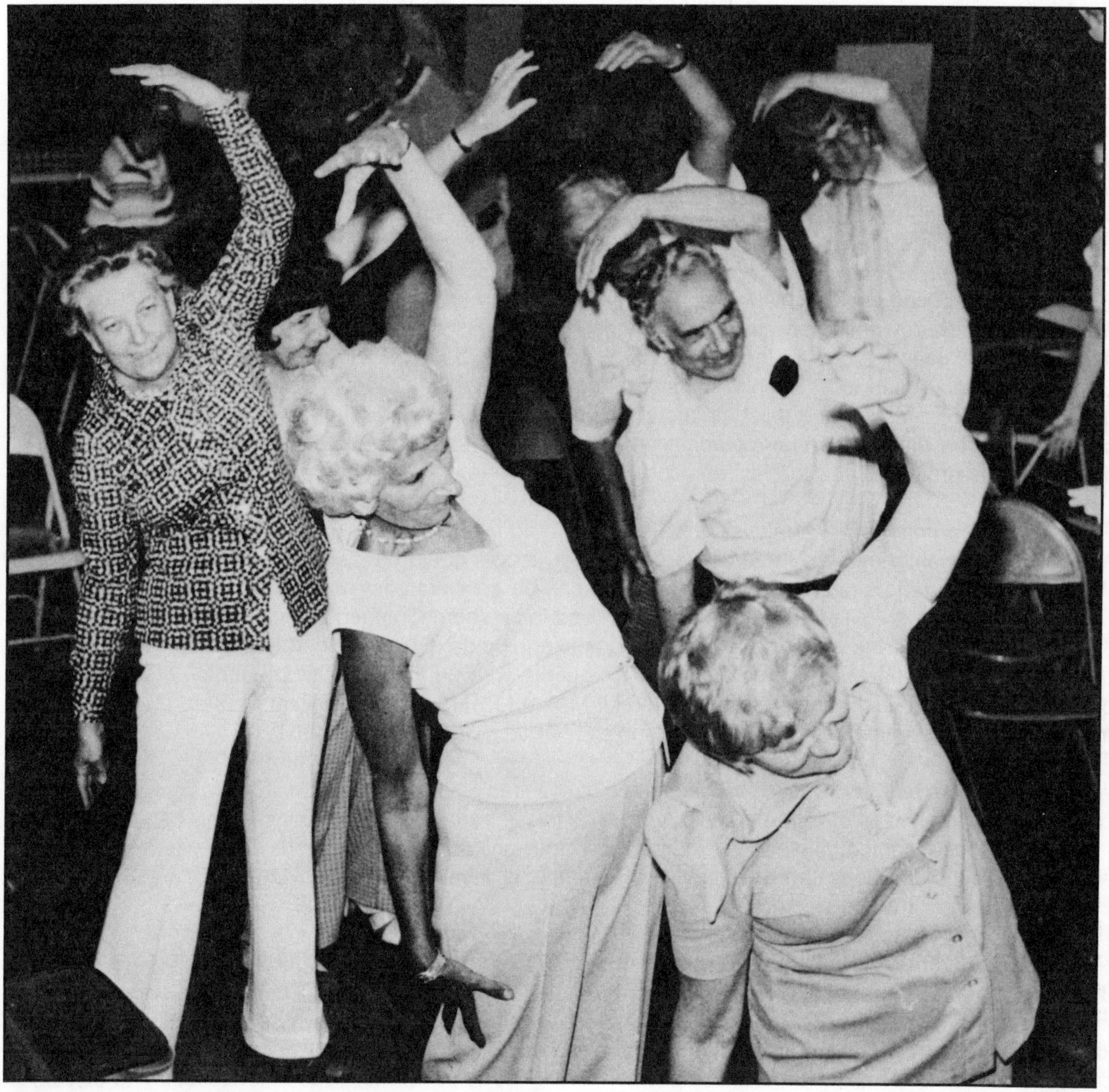

The warmup can be a time of creativity and variation.

The Aerobic Activity

The next 10-30 minutes of the class should involve continuous aerobic activity. A new group of exercisers may begin with as little as 5 minutes of aerobics, an easy walk as a rest, and then another few minutes of vigorous activity until endurance activity is improved. Depending on the entering fitness level of the participants, it my take months or years to reach 25-30 minutes at a training level of 65% or higher. Working for part of the time at 40% or slightly more of the maximal heart rate reserve and 10 minutes at a higher training level will result in small improvements in cardiorespiratory function over time until eventually a longer and more intense training period can be reached.

When working with people inexperienced with dance movement, it is best to include both rhythmic and non-rhythmic activities. The rhythmic activities can be any kind of locomotor pattern or dance step that uses the beat of the music and allows people to keep their heart rates at a training level. Dances in general need to be simple, or moderate tempo, have long repetitive phrases, a minimum of quick changes of direction and must be choreographed to allow for performance variations. Each group of people will be different in their coordination and ability to learn movement patterns. What may be simple for one group may be too fast and complex for another.

It is also important that elevation of feet off the floor be kept to a minimum. The typical hopping and jumping involved in aerobics for younger people could be disastrous for the older population. Joints often deteriorate with age and damage can be accelerated with an excess of jarring impact to those of the lower extremities. Therefore, dances need to be choreographed and planned in a sequence that constantly varies the type of stress to any one joint, avoids more than one hop or jump in a sequence, and gives the option of no elevation for people with particularly painful joints. Traditional folk dances such as the Russian Troika and the Israeli Mayim Mayim can be excellent for aerobics. Others may need to be modified because of their complexity or lack of aerobic potential.

One of the best approaches for endurance dance is to choreograph original dances suited to the preferences and abilities of a particular group. An endless variety of simple dances can be created using walking, easy jogging, skipping, waltzing, two-steps, polkas, and schottische patterns. For those with painful joints, the hops can be changed to knee lifts or eliminated, e.g., taking the hop out of a polka and making it a two-step.

To add variety to the class, dances should vary in formation between forward facing, circle dances without partners, circles with partners, partner dances back and forth across the floor, and free formations. The later are dances that allow the participant to move anywhere on the floor. These kinds of dances are helpful in developing the skills and coordination necessary to sense and then avoid collisions with other people. It also gives people the chance to cover more space if necessary to elevate their heart rates. The free formation is useful for introductory games like skipping about the room and circling elbows with people while learning their names.

Partner activities are an effective method of socializing the class. Circle partner dances such as the Troika or partner dances like the Virginia Reel develop a sense of unity, cooperation and interdependence among participants. Partner dances, because they are less vigorous, add to the social content of the class but they often, though not always, result in lower heart rates. On the other hand, two highly motivated partners may challenge each other to work harder than usual. A carefully planned class can counter a lowered heart rate from a partner dance by following with a more vigorous individual activity.

Dance can be as simple as varying between a two-step and a race walk or as complex as the Mayim Mayim. The complexity of the dances needs to be determined by the interests, rhythmic ability, and learning potential of individuals in the class. A careful balance must be achieved between those who need to feel the comfort and constant repetition of the same simple dances and those who like the challenge of more difficult variations.

Activities that do not rely on rhythm can be interspersed between dances. Various games or sport adaptations, circuit training activities, improvisations, etc., offer the non-dance oriented person a chance to move less self-consciously and often with more vigor. Any number of activities with playground balls can be a huge success. People are transported to their childhood as they learn to dribble, shoot baskets, throw and catch or kick the balls off the walls. Care must be taken to check heart rates often during these "play" periods to make sure heart rates are not exceeding a safe limit.

Improvisational ideas also work well in an endurance dance class. A great deal of laughter and work is accomplished by having people run or walk while leading with a particular body part, i.e. the nose, elbow, knee or backside. Mimicking various locomotor vehicles or making household chores larger than life can also be enjoyable and effective and give the participants a chance to contribute ideas for movement.

In addition to the socialization element of the class, offering a wide variety of activities appears to be the next most important criteria for maintaining compliance. There is no other age group that offers more variation between people in terms of interests, learning abilities, past experiences, fitness, and movement skills than the older population. Therefore, satisfying everyone takes a concentrated effort at providing variety. Building a large and varied repertoire of dances and activities is the first step. These can then be mixed and matched in different ways in each class, keeping the participants interested and guessing as to what is coming next. New dances will need to be repeated more often until mastered while older dances can be brought back when desired.

Dispersing dance music among many tapes rather than having the class set with one tape gives a great deal more freedom for the continuous creation of new and interesting class combinations. With this method, several tapes are usually needed for each class, including one for warmup music, a tape for each endurance dance or activity, another for cooldown, and music for the strength and flexibility exercises. Music can be acquired from many sources: the public library, record companies specializing in dance records, the radio, record stores, and most importantly, from the participants' own record collections.

Class planning must include ideas for smooth transitions between dances and continuous activity while tapes are being changed. Learning to move continuously is an unusual experience for the older adult. It usually takes a significant effort of coaching on the part of the instructor to keep the participants moving. Clever transition ideas and a great deal of encouragement of the participants are helpful. People must clearly understand that they must keep moving not only for a training effect but also to prevent blood from pooling in the lower extremities and causing dizziness or lightheadedness.

The Cooldown

A transition period between the endurance activity and rest is necessary to lower heart rate and body temperature gradually and to keep the blood from pooling. A simple walk with large arm movements is effective as a simple choreographed dance. Moving to time honored dances like the Greek Miserlou can produce a delightful sense of peace and relaxation after the vigor of aerobic activity. Playing with toys can also be an interesting cooldown. Examples include playing with gymnastic ribbons, slowly dribbling balls with the feet, or doing strengthening exercises with rubber tubing.

Strength and Flexibility Exercises

Endless variety can also be offered in this portion of the class. Exercises can be done standing using a chair as a "ballet barre," sitting in a chair or sitting or lying on the floor. For added interest, some of the exercises can be choreographed to music, but take care that the music and movement are at a comfortable tempo for the group. At other times, music can simply be used in the background. Dumbbells, wrist and ankle weights, or rubber tubing are a wonderful addition to this section of the class. Much more strength can be gained using these objects that simply using body weight.

This point in the program is also an excellent time to educate the class about proper alignment, the purpose and benefits of exercise, and safe and effective exercise techniques. Checking each other for proper alignment or technique can be a way of assuring they understand the points covered, providing more individual attention, and stimulating more interaction and , therefore, more socialization between participants.

Over time students need to learn intellectually as well as physically the "do's and don'ts" of exercise as we have learned in dance technique. The following is a list of some of these items. Although these recommendations appear "black and white," it should be noted that, like most things in life, there are gray areas. For example, while back arching may be hazardous to some people, others need back arching exercises because of their severely limited flexibility in this area. The best scenario is for the teachers to understand the kinesiological reasoning behind the "do's and don'ts" as well as the history and unique needs of each participant. With this knowledge, exercise variations can be prescribed as needed. For teachers who have not worked with this age group it is best to be conservative until the abilities of the group become clear.

DON'T	DO
1. Bounce to stretch	Teach people to stretch "quietly". Have them assume a position that stretches a particular muscle group and teach them to relax into the stretch.
2. Lock or hyperextend joints	Strengthening exercises for the muscles surrounding the joints. A dance teacher can help people become conscious of when they are hyperextending.
3. Throw the arms or legs	Control the motion. Teaching how to lengthen the limbs instead of throwing them into locked positions can be important in preventing injury.
4. Arch the back	Help people become conscious of their alignment and what they may need to correct. Specific exercise routines may need to be developed for individuals to do at home if progress is to be seen in class. These sequences will usually include strengthening exercises for the abdominals and back muscles and stretching exercises for the front of the shoulders.

DON'T (continued)	DO (continued)
5. Circle the head	Stretch the neck side to side and up and down. Dropping the head back could cut off circulation in the vertebral artery and aggravate cervical vertebrae.
6. Large torso circles or forward bends from the waist	Perform a roll of the spine with the knees bent and the abdominals active. Large movements of the torso without proper technique can be very injurious to the older adult with chronic back problems.
7. Allow the knees to bend in one direction and the feet to point in another	Keep knees and feet in alignment at all times to avoid twisting the knees. People need to be made conscious of where their knees are placed when bending at the knee. Often muscles need to be activated in ways to which the older adult is not accustomed.

Older adults will more quickly injure themselves or aggravate chronic problems than would a younger person. Particular attention should be paid in this section of the class to strengthening all major muscle groups. Strong muscles will help protect the joints from injury, give people the strength for daily chores and may also play a role in strengthening bone. These benefits are important for those older adults who have lost the strength to adequately care for themselves, and are at increased risk of bone fractures and/or those who experience weak and painful joints. Teaching the participants how to fall safely, lift heavy objects, and lower and rise from the floor can also be invaluable.

Following a strength exercise with a flexibility exercise for the same muscle group helps reduce after-exercise soreness and maintains range of motion while increasing strength. Exercises that increase flexibility can often reverse to some degree the loss of range of motion commonly seen in the older adult. In fact, research indicates that a great deal of this loss may be due to disuse and not just the aging process. Participants will excitedly relate the daily tasks they can easily perform once again with their improved range of motion.

Ending class with stretching and relaxation exercises and techniques can be helpful for the older adult. Many people have difficulty sleeping as they grow older and benefit from learning relaxation techniques. Participants will leave class relaxed, feeling good, and thoroughly cooled down.

Additional Safety Precautions

Reducing stress to the joints requires proper footwear and floor constitution. Participants need education as to the kinds of exercise shoes available and the pros and cons of each type. Running, court or aerobic dance shoes can all be appropriate for the endurance dance class. Shoes must be chosen according to the problems and/or requirements of the individual. People should be encouraged to go to a reputable athletic shoe store with knowledgeable sales people to help them choose the best shoe for their needs. The importance of good footwear must be emphasized to the older adult who may not be comfortable or familiar with the cost or benefits of athletic shoes.

A sprung wood floor is the most shock absorbent type of floor and therefore the best for endurance dance. Although padding or rugs would appear to offer more cushioning, the loss of foot stability with impact can quickly lead to injury in the ankle, knee, or hip. The most ideal situation is a large gymnasium with a high ceiling. This not only provides a sprung wood floor but also the advantage of the ceiling height which allows the use of balls and other such toys in the class. Older adults often suffer poor eyesight, hearing loss and a decline in their body's ability to regulate temperature. Thus the exercise space needs to be well lit, ventilated and/or heated adequately and acoustically sound.

Limiting the class to a total of 20-24 participants is also an important safety precaution. The potential for health problems or injury is somewhat greater with an older population, and instructors constantly need to monitor the performance of the participants. Anyone teaching a class of this nature _must_ be CPR certified and knowledgeable of emergency procedures should a situation arise.

Dancing has weathered centuries as one of man's favorite pastimes. With this in mind, it is no surprise that an endurance exercise class based on rhythmic movement will be so successful. Utilizing ideas from all the dance forms to create a total fitness package not only gives variety but caters to the whole person. Participants have the potential of improving strength, flexibility, and endurance as well as their balance, coordination, body image, self-image and socialization skills. In addition, their experience with movement will better help them appreciate the art of dance and turn them on to the many possibilities of the social forms of dance. When dancers share their joy of movement with a new audience it furthers the cause of dance and all involved benefit.

REFERENCES

Agre, J.C., Smith, E.L., Pierce, L.E., McAdam, M., & Raab, D.M. (in press). Light resistance and stretching exercise in elderly women: effects upon strength. _Archives of Physical Medicine and Rehabilitation._

Brody, J.A. & Brock, D.B. (1985). Epidemiologic and statistical characteristics of the United States elderly population. In C. E. Finch & E. L. Schneider (Eds.), _Handbook of the Biology of Aging, Second Edition._ New York: Van Nostrand Reinhold.

Garrick, J.G., Gillien, D.M., & Whiteside, P. (1986). The epidemiology of aerobic dance injuries. _The American Journal of Sports Medicine, 14,_(1), 67-72.

McArdle, W.D., Katch, F.I., & Katch, V.L., (1981). _Exercise Physiology: Energy, Nutrition, and Human Performance_. Philadelphia: Lea & Fabiger.

National Institutes of Health, Consensus Development Conference on Osteoporosis, (1984). Washington, D.C: NIH.

Pollock, M.L., Wilmore, J.H., & Smith, E.L. (1978). _Health and Fitness Through Physical Activity._ New York: John Wiley.

Raab, D.M., Agre, J.C., McAdam, M., & Smith, E.L. (in press). Light resistance and stretching exercise in elderly women: effects upon flexibility. Archives of Physical Medicine and Rehabilitation.

Richie, D.H., Kelso, S.F., & Bellucci, P.A. (1985). Aerobic dance injuries: A retrospective study of instructors and participants. The Physician and Sportsmedicine, 13(2), 130-140.

Shephard, R.J. Physical Activity and Aging. (1978). London: Croom Helm.

Smith, E.L. (1984). Special considerations in developing exercise programs for the older adult. In J.D. Matarazzo, N.E. Miller, S.M. Weiss, J.A. Herd & S.M. Weiss (Eds.), Behavioral Health: A Handbook of Health Enhancement and Disease Prevention. New York: John Wiley, 526-546.

Smith, E.L. & Gilligan, C. (1987). Inactivity and exercise effects on bone. The Physician and Sportsmedicine, 15(11).

Smith, E.L. & Raab, D.M. (1986). Osteoporosis and physical activity. In P.O. Astrand & G. Grimby (Eds.), Physical Activity in Health and Disease. Stockholm: Amqvist & I, 149-156.

Topics in Geriatric Rehabilitation.(1985). 1(1).

Vetter, W.L., Helfet, D.L., Spear, K., & Matthews, L.S. (1985). Aerobic dance injuries. The Physician and Sportsmedicine, 13(2), 114-120.

6

Benefits of Dance in the Process of Aging and Retirement for the Older Adult

Sherrill Berryman-Miller

Introduction

With the older population ranging from ages 65 to over 85, growing at a much more rapid rate than it has during previous decades, there has become a demand to address their needs of total well-being and longevity of life. In the article "Camping It Up With Seniors" Dan Leviton, founder and director of Adults, Health and Developmental Program at the University of Maryland refers to physical fitness as one of the variables that can be used to predict life satisfaction. The stagnation or decline in physical activity is particularly evident as people grow older. There is an inactivity of muscles and joints, improper breathing and slower, laborious movements of the body-as-a-whole. For formal and informal health practitioners interested in the ways that dance movement can be used as a form of physical exercise, this article delineates several programs using dance with the older adult experiencing the life changes of aging and retirement. The range of physical and intellectual stimulation possible in dance sessions indicates that this art form can serve the biological and social needs of the older adult while promoting the quality of life.

Paradoxically, one may spend a lifetime of striving for comfort in old age, only to discover that once simple activities such as getting out of bed, walking, climbing stairs, and entering a car have become labored but valued assets in surviving with comfort and pleasure. The pursuit of these activities takes on new signif-

---

Reprinted with permission from Activities, Adaptation & Aging, Vol. 9(1), Fall 1986

icance in the latter part of life when many of the other components of life or role activities are curtailed. The research by Penny La Roque et al. observed that:

> Increasingly, we use elevators or escalators instead of stairs, ride instead of walk and only expeience athletic endeavors vicariously. Flexibility, strength and cardiovascular fitness decline steadily. As a result of this inactivity, joint action decreases, ligaments tighten and muscles lose tone. Many older persons suffer from aches and pains which could be directly related to their sedentary life style. (1983, p. 77)

The value of regular participation in exercise programs can help retard this physical deterioration that occurs with aging and inactivity. Dance therapist, Erna Caplow Lindner, points out that:

> The great range of physical and intellectual stimulation possible in dance sessions, whether in therapy, recreation or educational settings, indicates that this art form holds much promise in helping older adults experience a greater sense of oneness with others, improved self-esteem and communication, and an overall sense of physical well-being. (1982, p.167)

Understanding that dance in all manifestations can be a lifetime activity the therapeutic, psychosocial, and recreational value has been growing among dance and physical educators, recreation leaders, and health professionals such as physical therapists (Pruett, 1983).

The Biological Nature Of Aging and the Social Nature of Retirement

During the 1960s and '70s research in the universities and public agencies reflected an increased attempt to understand the biological nature of aging and the social nature of retirement. Evidence from the Association of American Medical Colleges 1983 Proceedings of the Regional Institutes of Geriatrics and Medical Education concluded that the biological aging process is not only affected by the lifestyle change of retirement but also educational levels, nutrition, self-care, economic status, family relationships and other social, and physical aspects of health in the middle and later life cycles. This biopsychosocial process is being studied and analyzed to organize a national effort to expand the quality of life for the nation's elderly by linking research to practice. Biologists, sociologists, and psychologists have developed a new language and new ideas around the study of gerontology--the science dealing with aging and the special problems of older people.

The terms "biological aging" and "biological clock" changed the scientific measurement of human aging (Garnet, 1982). Today people age not according to their number of birthdays but according to their physical conditions. At a 1984 conference on "The Multi-Facet Roles of Dance and the Elderly" held at New York University, Dr. Michael L. Freedman, Director of Geriatric Medicine, New York University referred to incompetence, incontinence, impaired homeostatis, immobility and iatrogenic diseases as areas of concern for the over 65 population when there is a decline in health maintenance and physical activity. The words "biological clock" suggests that a person is as old as his or her biological resources--arteries or spine or any other organ system dictates. A person of any age with advanced cardiovascular diseasee is "older" than a person of seventy who is free of this ailment.

Closely related to biological concepts of aging is the concept of senescence. Senescence is the stage of life that everyone hopes to last longer than infancy, childhood, and adolescence put together. Gerontologists found that the happiness or unhappiness that people experienced during retirement was determined not only by circumstances but also by beliefs and attitudes relating to work and senescence. Scott H. Beck (1982) found that although a negative bivariate relationship exists between retirement and happiness with life, retirement had no significant net effect. Health was found to be one of the factors having a greater impact on life safistaction.

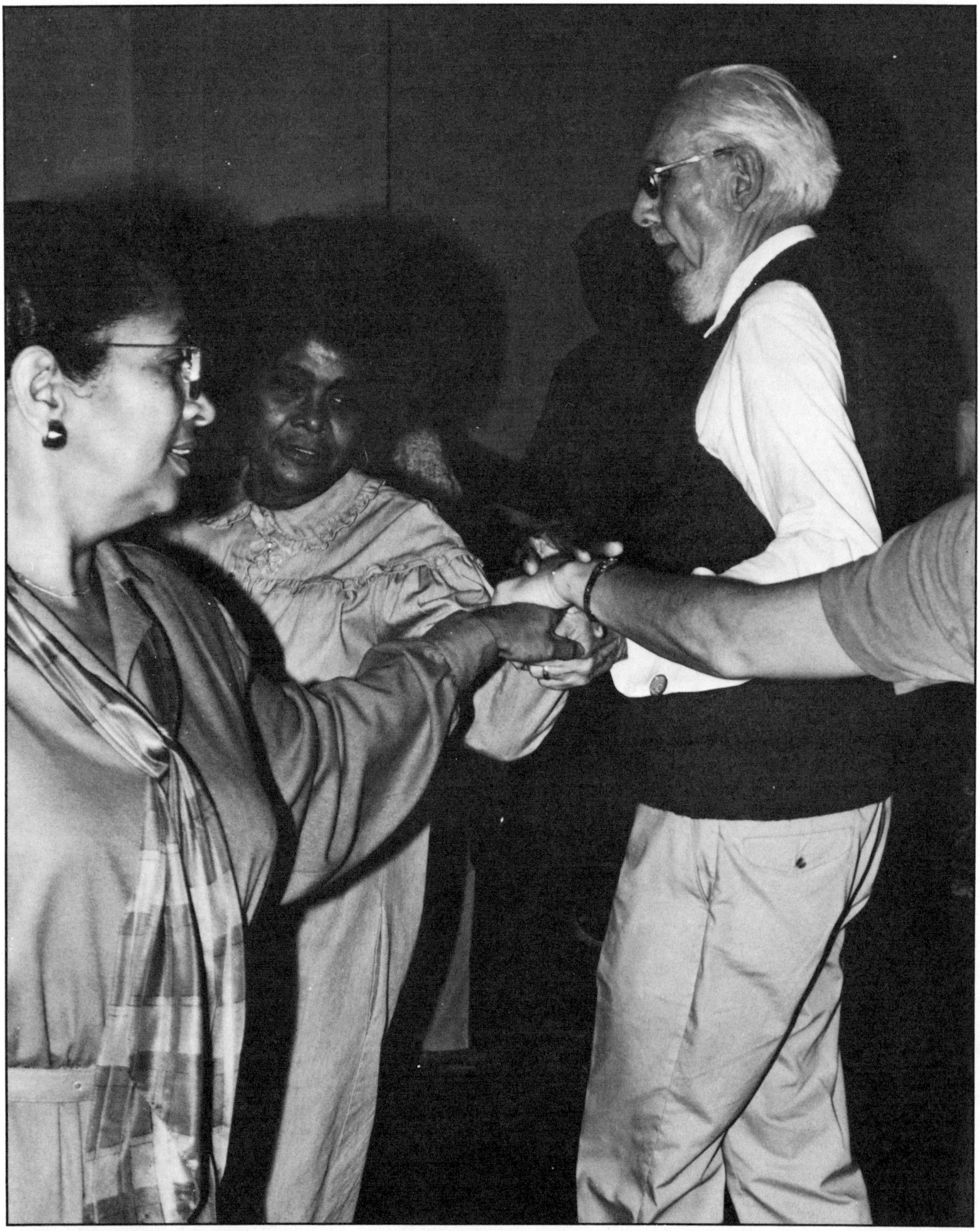

PHOTO COURTESY OF ANDRE RICHARDSON

Older adults need an opportunity to participate with their peers in meaningful activities.

Though retirement means cessatoin of employment, it does not bring to an end the belief that work is an expression of usefullness, meaningfulness, and status. In Eva Garnet's *Movement is Life* the anthropologist Margaret M. Clark (1968) wrote:

> Such values as youth activity, multiple role involvement and independence as well as productivity, are adverse to aging changes. Daily, we see the personal tragedies resulting from the contradiction between the contemporary needs of the elderly and these archaic attitudes towards a meaningful life. (1982, p. 4)

Older people need an incentive to restructure their lives after retirement. They need an opportunity to participate with their peers in meaningful activities and ways that are validated by society. In the classic article "The Life Course of Individuals," J. A. Clausen writes:

> Physical and social psychological development interact in a social matrix made up of group memeberships and of shared or conflicting expectations that bind men to each other or divide them and that contribute crucially to the individual's own identity. What an individual is at any given time--what goals he pursues, what meanings events have for him, how he relates to others, and how others view him--depends upon the complex sequence of interactions among the influences upon him and the patterns that he himself has evolved for coping with his world. (1972, p. 42)

Physical fitness can be an integral part of life's design for a more satisfying life in senescence (Garnet, 1982).

Methods of Dealing with the Sedentary Life-Style After Retirement

Although western society has always valued work as spiritually desirable and leisure as spiritually suspect, life after retirement can occur with an effective and efficient method of dealing with the sedentary life-style prevalent today in this technologically advanced society.

The 1984 conference on the "Multi-Facet Role of Dance and the Elderly," co-sponsored by the Dance Department of New York University and the National Dance Association presented a variety of approaches being utilized with the older adult in keeping their minds and bodies active when many of the other components of life or role activities are curtailed. These approaches involve the art form of dance, combine affective and cognitive learning, and stimulate participant creativity. Chapter 24, which includes a listing of dance artists, educators, and therapists, and their methods of exploring dance for the older adult, may be useful as a resorce for further contact and guidance of how to integrate the physical activity of dance in the life of an older adult who encounters a decrease in movement as he/she approaches retirement age.

While participation in a well-designed dance program can be beneficial, participation in a poor one is dangerous. Exercise of an inappropriate type, duration, intensity, frequency, and progression can trigger a cardiovascular accident or serious musculoskeletal injury (Lopez, 1983). The American Alliance Committee on Aging has established guidelines that should be an integral part of any instructor's program that will involve the older adults of our society.

1. Each participant should have a medical examination prior to beginning an exercise program, prefereably by a physician with knowledge in exercise physiology and the values and risks of regular exercise for the older adult.

2. Each participant's physiological capacity should be the key to planning the type, intensity, duration, frequency, and progression of exercise program.

3. Each participant should have access to a well-defined emergency plan which includes an instructor with training in cardio-pulmonary resuscitation techniques.

Although the aging process is multifactorial and will result in greater susceptibility to disease, the human being does have the capability to live to be 100 years old with exercise as the cornerstone to a healthy and functional life--physically, socially, psychologically and spiritually.

Though retirement can become a depersonalized, uninteresting stage of adult development where one can feel removed from the reality of the adult's environment, the older adult can achieve more in these later years of life by finding joy in movement.

If we are to be effective with this growing population which by the year 2000 will have 20% over the age of 65, increasing the knowledge of everyone who will eventually be an older adult is essential.

REFERENCES

A Synopsis of the Conference on The Multi-Faceted Roles of Dance on the Older Adult. New York, December 8, 1984. National dance Association and New York University.

Alliance Committee on Aging. Guidelines for Exercise Programs for Older Adults. Reston, Virginia, 1981.

Beck, Scott H. 1982. Adjustment to and satisfactoin with retirement. *Journal of Gerontology,* 37, 5, 602-603.

Boscov, Rema. "Camping It Up With Seniors." Washington Post Style Plus. April 19, 1985, p. C5.

Clark, Margaret M. 1968. The anthropology of aging: A new area for studies of culture and personality. In Bernice L. Neugarten (Ed.), *Middle Age and Aging* (pp. 433-443). Chicago: University of Chicago Press.

Clausen, J. A. "The Life Course of Individuals," quoted in *Movement is Life*, Eva D. Garnet. Princeton, New Jersey: Princeton Book Co. 1982.

Garnet, Eva D. 1982. Movement is Life. Princeton, New Jersey: Princeton Book Co.

LaRocque, Penny & Campagna, P. D. 1983. Physical Activity Through Rhythmic Exercise for Elderly Persons Living in a Senior Citizen Residence. *Activities, Adaptation & Aging*, 4(1), 77-81.

Lindner, Erna D. 1982. Dance as therapeutic invention for the elderly. *Educational Gerontology*, 8, 6, 167-173.

Lopez, Richard. 1983. Guidelines for using dance with older adults. *Journal of Physical Education, Health, Recreation and Dance*, 45, 5, 43-51.

Proceedings of the Regional Institutes on Geriatrics and Medical Education. 1982. Washington, D.C.: Association of American Medical Colleges.

Pruett, Diane M. 1983. Dance for the older adult. *Journal of Physical Education, Health, Recreation and Dance,* 45, 5, 43-51.

II. Program Models

7

Movement Activities for Older Adults

Bernadette Hecox

It is generally agreed that as one gets older both exercising and keeping up with social activities contribute toward maintaining a vital life-style. Participating in a movement/dance group is a delightful way to do both.

Conducting such groups for "swinggin' seniors" at community centers, for patients in long-term hospitals, or for residents in nursing homes can be fun, rewarding and challenging. It's fun sharing good times with the participants. It's rewarding seeing someone walk with strides instead of dragging steps or get out of a chair more easily and hearing participants say, "Please come back tomorrow. I feel so good after class." The challenge to group leaders is to plan appropriate classes and to put their all into each session. The method to help leaders meet the challenge presented here is based on one developed for creative modern dance classes and adapted for older adults.

The philosophy underlying this approach is to think holistically. A movement group implies that the activities are directed toward the physical parameter of the "person". However, if and how people move is based as much on their psychological and social needs and strengths as on their body. Attending sessions where one is looked at and spoken to directly, called by name, and sometimes praised, encourages enthusiastic participation. Boring movements done repeatedly, or difficult movements which make one feel fearful or defeated, discourage participation. Thus, it is essential that the psychological, social and physical effects can be considered for each activity.

Organizing Groups

Successful groups may have four or twenty-four members depending on their physical and mental health and on the number of assistants available. Groups of five to ten disabled people require at least one person assisting. Unless the group is small, one and one-half hour sessions are recommended. This allows for 15 minutes to get everyone organized, one full hour for activities including rest periods and "chatting" now and then, and 15 minutes to clean up and write progress reports.

Select participants with caution. Older people may be limited by high blood pressure, cardiac problems, or arthritis. Written approval from a physician should mention any precautions to be observed or activities to be avoided. Leaders not qualified to understand these precautions should team up with a health professional.

Planning Activities

Each session must be carefully planned. At first this may take over an hour. Later, much less time is needed. Well-rounded classes should include warm-up periods, rest times, a variety of activities, and at least one important "high point."

First, set goals. If the primary goal is to maintain or improve physical abilities, activities may be directed toward relaxation, flexibility, muscle strengthening, breathing improvement, endurance, balance, coordination and ambulation activities. But think holistically! Add components to make each activity a positive psychological, social experience. If the primary goal is fun, make it physically beneficial as well.

One activity may address many goals. For example having the entire group hold hands, swaying and swinging arms while singing a familiar song, integrates exercises for breathing, voice articulation, range of arm motion, and standing balance. Additionally, touching others and recalling pleasant memories evoked by the song may support the psychological/social parameters which in turn, encourages fuller participation in the physical activity.

Each session, designed specifically for the group, should be a creative experience for both the leader and the participants. Although three different groups may all need exercises to decrease "stiffness" in the knees, one group may tend to enjoy fun and mental challenges. They might learn a knee flexion-extension exercise with rhythmical time changes using various arm and leg movements and a seated Rockette Kick routine. Another group might be more artistic and creative. They might improvise to discover how many ways in what positions each can straighten and bend knees--standing, sitting, lying on backs--no two people doing quite the same thing. Adding a beginning and end to the improvised movements creates a brief composition which can be performed for the group. A third group may be more interested in games. Teams could kick a light-weight ball to each other using the legs or a balloon may be passed from one person to another sitting in a circle. Occasionally, all three groups may appreciate doing traditional knee exercises.

Leaders should encourage participants to create movements and to contribute ideas. The leader may present a simple movement and ask participants to suggest variations. Once they learn to share ideas, the unusual movements they create themselves may be more effective and fun than those devised by the leaders.

To develop the "free thinking" needed to plan holistic, creative experiences, consider the many components of movement, rather than traditional exercises.

Movement Components

What moves? Here consider the *physical* parameters of a "person." Decide what the group's physical strengths and/or needs may be and what special attention certain people may require. For example, the entire group may need to improve balance and can practice shifting weight from side to side with music. Mr. B. can do it independently so should be given plenty of open space to enjoy it, but Mrs. L. will need a walker, so one must be available.

Where does this body move? Consider the spatial areas in which the body moves, the levels, planes, and directions. Awareness of movement occurring *within* the body, how the movement "feels," as well as how it is moving in the space surrounding it should be developed. Use the space as close to and as far from the body as one can reach, and the space beyond reach. Verbal suggestions such as "touch the ceiling," or "move your leg very close to the chair and then as far from it as possible" emphasize spatial as well as body awareness. This reinforces what occurs in daily activities; people think "*bend down*" and "*reach up*" as

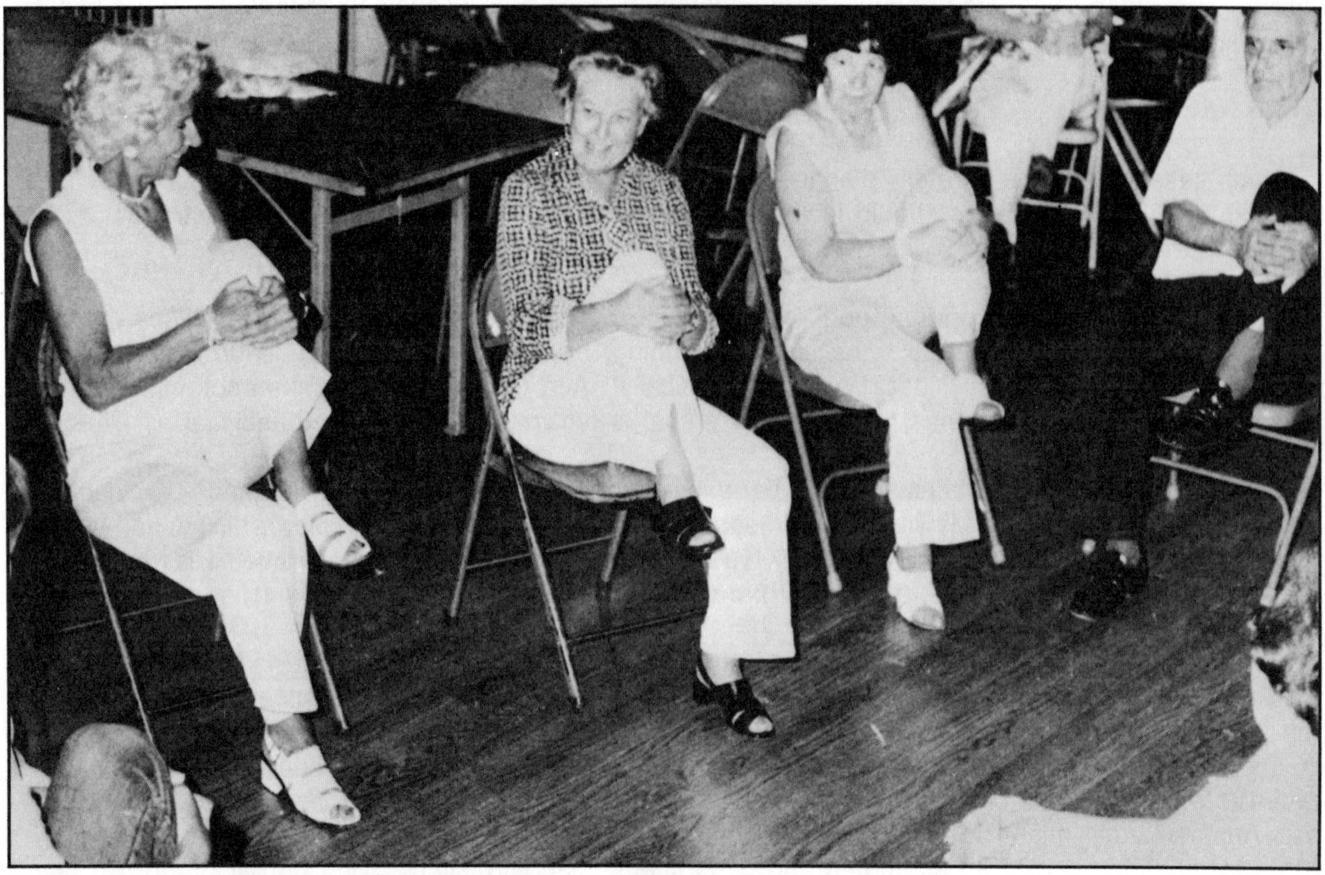

A comfortable group feeling can be encouraged when everyone, including the leader, is seated in a circle.

much as *"bend the back"* or *"lift the arm."*

An entire session spent sitting or standing in one spot facing forward, or moving only in a forward direction is dull and deprives participants of functional movement experiences. Vary exercises by including a turning component or a stretch sidewards or backwards while looking in those directions.

When people confined to wheelchairs are pushed through space in many directions and circles, and the person seated in the chair thinks, reaches, and focuses out in the direction the chair is moving, they experience a great feeling of penetrating space.

With older adults, major emphasis should be on outside space, people, and objects rather than "center" awareness. It helps draw them "out of self" and distracts them from pain and worry. References to objects or space dealing with functions, such as "step toward the TV knob" or "shake hands with your neighbor" are helpful.

How does the body move? It is useful to apply Rudolph Laban's concepts when considering how the body moves. Each person's movements are a unique combination of timing, use of space, force, and flow qualities. Sometimes, they are not the most efficient for a function. If the goal is to change a person's movement qualities for more effective daily living (for example, for quicker movement), movements should begin with the speed which is comfortable for that person. Then proceed to the contrasts within that person's range, from the quickest to the slowest he can comfortably move. This gradually expands the range so results come without forcing someone to move in an unnatural way.

Assume that a whole group is extremely tense one day. Rather than saying, "Relax, relax," start with a tension exercise such as, "Make fists like a boxer--open those fingers as if they were *shooting* out, now let them hang limp." Later introduce activities using a more relaxing tone of voice, mellow music, and perhaps movements incorporating Laban's "floating" quality.

Always use the principle of starting where participants are comfortable. Although the goal may be for people to be able to touch the floor, if they *cannot* do it, begin by asking only to "touch the knees." Later change this to "touch the ankles" and, when that is achieved, ask them to "touch the floor." A leader can achieve the same goals without frustrating anyone.

When and with whom do we move? There are times when it is desirable to be concentrating on "self" and times when it is good to get one "out of self." Group activities depend upon sensitive use of interpersonal and spatial relationships.

When everyone, including the leader, is seated in a circle, a comfortable group feeling is encouraged. In this position each person is placed equally and can see everyone else. When each is given as much personal space as possible scattered about the room, "self" involvement is encouraged. This may help participants to discover "how a movement feels" or to create movements. Positioning participants in rows facing the leader standing in front draws attention to the leader and is useful when striving to teach important points. Working with partners or in groups of three is an easy way to develop interpersonal relationships and to share ideas. Large groups may be intimidating for these purposes. It is valuable to use *many different* spatial and interpersonal relationships during every session.

Why do we move? Motivation cannot be overemphasized. Older adults are likely to participate in activities that are fun, satisfying, reduce pain, evoke artistic or spiritual responses, stimulate pleasurable social involvement, or provide physical or intellectual challenges. Use imagery. "Let your body move like a piece of limp spaghetti." Use fantasy. Instead of asking someone to do an arm exercise ten times, "Pretend you are a World Series pitcher--Wind Up! Pitch! Strike One!" Next time, "Ball One," for as many repetitions as you wish. Then, to use the other arm, become a left-handed pitcher. Movement games and simple variations of ballroom or ethnic dances help people relate to other people.

Objects and props can be useful. It is easier to walk around a real chair than an imaginary one as a reference point is helpful. "Reach and look toward the window." "Slide sidewards through the doorway." Doing movements with scarves, flowers, and lightweight balls can make otherwise repetitious movement fun.

Use music and other sounds. Music can be magical, and can inspire people to move. Most people respond to some form of music, classical, ethnic, spiritual, pop. Lawrence Welk appeals to many. Use music that both the leader and the participants can enjoy, but use it carefully. Persons with Parkinson's Disease or arthritis may have a wonderful sense of rhythm, but if they cannot keep in time because of a disability, they will become frustrated and may not move at all. Playing music constantly may diminish its effectiveness. It may be appreciated more if used only for portions of a session. Silence, voice sounds, cymbals, drum beats, and hands clapping can all be effective if not overused.

The proper ambience for each activity also motivates. Soft lights, a low voice and soft music encourages relaxation; a louder voice and upbeat music inspires exciting movements. Either for an entire session can be an overload. Probably the attitude of the leader is the one most important factor for successful movement groups. It takes a few sessions to develop intergrated groups, so leaders should not be discouraged if the first few sessions are not ideal. They continue to grow and get better with time. If the performer "gives" and the audience "responds," the performer gives more and gets more response. For both the participants and the leaders the entire "person" is enriched.

8

Adaptation Of Social And Popular Dances For The Elderly

Erna Caplow Lindner and Leah Harpaz

Dance specialists and physical educators who work with older adults are increasingly aware of the important role that social and popular dances can play in enhancing the pleasure and physical status of the participants. The diversity of these dances offers possibilities for vigorous as well as less taxing activity which may provide stimulation and produce improved mobility, coordination, and range of motion. Sometimes authentic versions of folk and ballroom dances are quite intricate and challenging for people with physical or mental limitations. However, with careful planning and modifications, the ever increasing number of elderly people in our society can enjoy this valuable resource.

Values of Dance for the Elderly

Through the physical, social, and creative elements of dance it is possible to involve both healthy and disabled older adults in meaningful programs. The nonverbal, rhythmic character of dance makes it appropriate and even basically appealing to aged people who may have sensory deficits such as those involving sight, hearing, and speech. Results show that, through the medium of movement, one can even overcome difficulties with comprehension (Bright, 1972; Helm & Gill, 1975; Merritt, 1971).

Furthermore, dance offers the potential to enhance an individual's self-image and to provide the opportunity for pleasurable sharing which may overcome the loneliness of advanced years. This sense of isolation, which is so common as we grow older, can be relieved through group dancing which develops a feeling of community (Bartenieff, 1972; Irwin, 1972; Rose, 1974). Shared movement experiences help to establish trust and confidence for more meaningful relationships with others. Berger and Berger, (1973), Goldberg & Fitzpatrick (1980), Hecox, Levine & Scott (1976), Lemon (1972), and Schoenfeld (1977) have all documented the successful application of dance activity as recreation and therapy in programs for the elderly. The increased participation, improved modes of interaction and higher levels of self-esteem have proved to be of utmost importance to the general well-being of aging individuals, as reported by participants, staff, peers, and medical personnel in the open community and in institutions (Lindner, Harpaz & Samberg, 1979; Samuels, 1973)

Uniquely Appropriate Characteristics of Social and Popular Dances

The use of social and popular dances is especially effective with geriatric groups because, in addition to providing physical activity, they are a normal social expression. The dances have the potential for direct application at community and family gatherings. Social dancing relates to the psychosocial experiences of the individual. People respond more easily and naturally to movement patterns that are familiar to them. Older adults between the ages of sixty-five and ninety are products of the "touch" dancing era, rather than the independent styles of contemporary rock and disco.

In addition, there is the possibility of an improved sense of personal identity through activity that utilizes the individual's ethnic and cultural idioms (Boxberger & Cotter, 1968; Layman, 1960). When a leader utilizes the music and dances from this heritage it evokes a physical, mental and emotional response from the participants. The dances and songs that were popular when one was a young adult, strong and full of hopes and dreams, are the ones that are recognized and welcomed by the elderly. They assist in recalling proud accomplishments, tender moments and even significant insights which may make the present more acceptable (Butler, 1963; Sandel, 1978).

Another important aspect of the social dances, relative to the older population, is the necessary interdependence involved in holding onto one another. This supportive physical contact provided by dancing with someone in a close position is pleasant and rewarding. Within the relaxed atmosphere of a dance session, each person can be offered an opportunity to enjoy being accepted and can participate as part of a couple or a group.

The dynamics and style of social dancing also present an acceptable outlet for healthy and appropriate sexuality. Dance group members enthusiastically respond to sensuous, provocative rhythms. For example, it is enjoyable to continue to be recognized as a sexual being and to be encouraged to react in familiar "feminine" or "masculine" body language in response to Tangos, Rhumbas, or Greek Syrtos.

Folk and ballroom dances provide the security of familiar steps and patterns. The simple, repetitive form offers safety, ritual power, and pleasant memory recall. Often the repeated movement sequences produce memory stimulation and cognitive responses with great therapeutic affect. The arranged patterning of folk dances also may be welcomed by many aged persons who are accustomed to an environment which has been more formal and restrictive than the "do your own thing" culture of today. Group members find it easier to create their own modifications and additions to a basic dance form.

The other characteristic of social and popular dances such as: action patterns involving a variety of body parts, strong rhythmic sequences, and well-defined structure make them comparatively simple to teach and perform. Therefore, the elderly person will be able to derive feelings of satisfaction and accomplishment from participating in this type of dancing.

Necessary Modifications

Many dance patterns need to be modified because they are too long, physically taxing, or inappropriate to a particular place or group. But, when changes are made, care must be taken to retain the original essence of the dance so that it is still valid and relevant for the participants. Sometimes the steps or space patterns are too complicated or overly vigorous for the aged. The disabilities common to older people can limit their movement responses. Thus, it is helpful to simplify the dance or

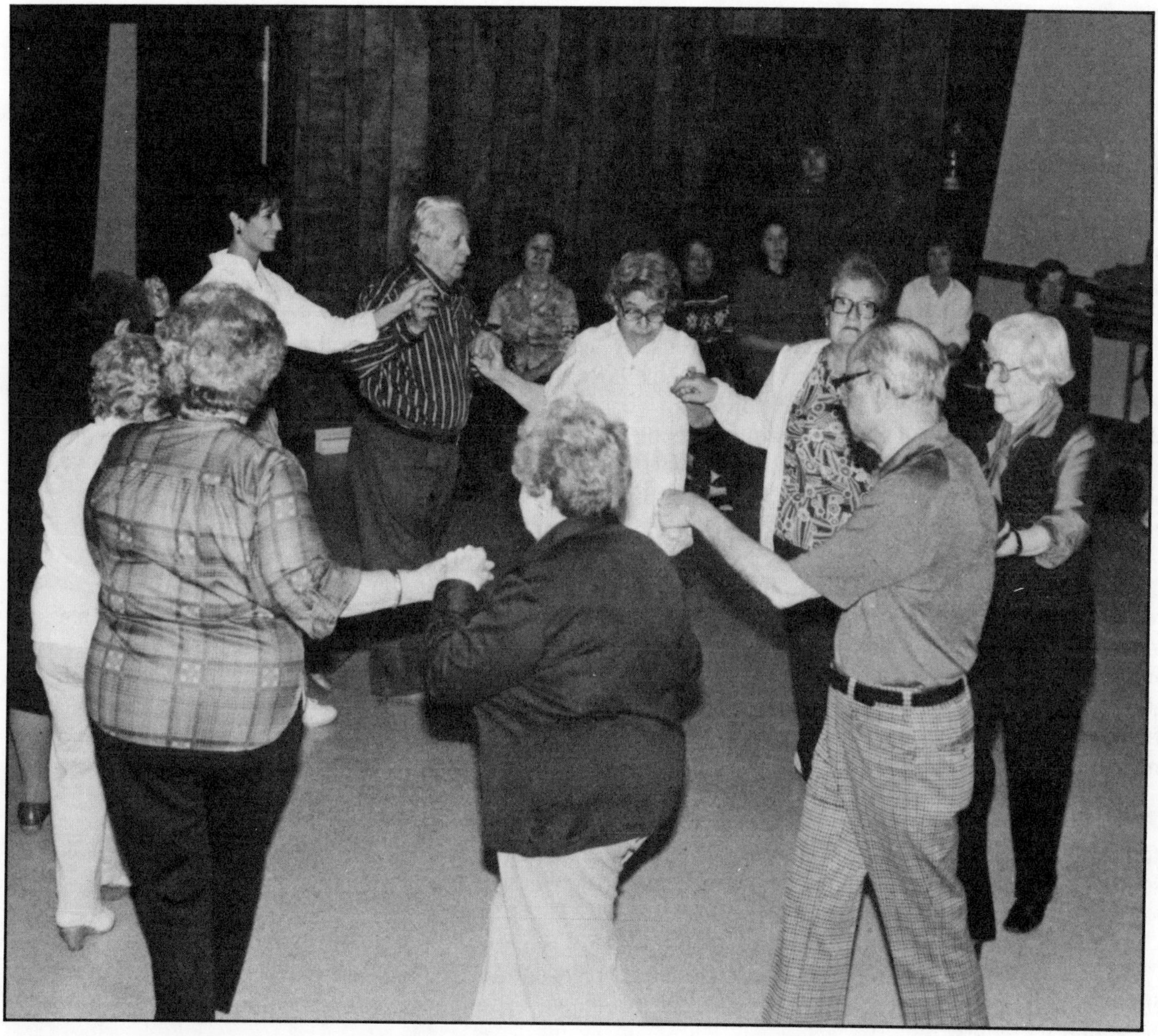

PHOTO COURTESY OF DAVID E. CORBIN

The "Silver Streak Dancers" of the Jewish Community Center, Kansas City, enjoy the social aspects of dance.

make modifications that change the original emphasis on footwork to the use of torso or arm movements. Dances can also be changed so that they are done only to one side, with just one body part, in a limited space with minimal motion, or at a much slower tempo. Decreased vision and hearing may also necessitate simple and extremely clear directions. Sometimes singing or saying what is done as the dance progresses can be fun as well as a good learning device. The "Alley Cat" is a good example of a dance that the group can "sing along" as they move: "out-in, out-in, back-close, knee, knee, clap and turn" while the music plays.

Most elderly groups consist of more women than men. Therefore, partner dances may be more acceptable if they are rearranged for single dancers in lines or circles. Circle and line formations can help participants follow the dance sequences as they watch each other. These formations also add a sense of security through group unity in action. However, no matter what spatial arrangement the dance may ultimately be performed in, the dancers are ideally arranged in lines facing the leader during the teaching of dances that have specific steps. This is so that they can follow the demonstration accurately. In many dances, the participants do not have to conform to exact instructions regarding which foot or side to use. They are just encouraged to respond to the rhythm and the general form of the movement phrase. But when a dance travels progressively in a circle or when it is necessary to coordinate one's actions with others, then the leader will find it useful to encourage the performance of specific foot patterns and directional cues.

The memory spans of the elderly may be short and so a leader can not have expectations of conscious carryover from one session to the next. Thus, a review is essential for each activity. This repetition may help to develop an adequate level of proficiency which will then produce feelings of improved self-confidence. Dances should be altered to include only a few different steps that are repeated and can be learned, preferably, within one session. For example, with some groups the "Miserlou" is taught as a dance with only one simple version of the grapevine step which is repeated throughout the music. Then, after this part has been mastered, other elements of the original dance may be introduced.

Leaders of geriatric groups may modify social and popular dances so that non-ambulatory participants can dance either in their chairs or while holding on to their walkers or canes. Even hat and cane dances may be arranged to incorporate an authentic cane or crutch in the choreography (Hill, 1976; Lindner, Harpaz and Samberg, 1977).

Considerations of the intellectual alertness, physical ability, and emotional status of the dancers help to guide the leader in the selection of movement experiences that are potentially satisfying for the group members.

Guidelines for Adaptation

Music that is selected for elderly groups, whether active or limited, will be most suitable if it can be adjusted to the preferences of the participants by utilizing a phonograph that has tone, volume, and tempo controls. A variety of lively selections that are easily followed, obviously recognizable and clearly repeated will encourage a wide range of responses from even depressed or lethargic groups.

It is helpful to select dances with brief step sequences. Dances that do not require very quick reaction responses or different level changes will be most successful with people who are not in prime physical condition. Structure that is supportive, but not restrictive, has the most value for these groups.

CRITERIA FOR MUSIC SELECTION

1. SIMPLE RHYTHMIC STRUCTURE
2. SHORT MELODIC PHRASES
3. MODERATE TEMPOS
4. STRONGLY ACCENTED SELECTIONS
5. FAMILIAR MELODIES OR STYLES
6. MELLOW SOUND QUALITY
7. VARIETY OF RHYTHMS AND FORM

GUIDELINES FOR ADAPTING DANCES

1. FOLLOW DOMINANT MUSIC ACCENTS
2. CREATE BRIEF MOVEMENT SEQUENCES
3. UTILIZE SIMPLE STEPS & SLOW, EASY TURNS
4. LIMIT MOTION PRIMARILY TO ONE LEVEL
5. INCORPORATTE EASY BALANCING & SLOW DIRECTIONAL CHANGES
6. PROVIDE APPROPRIATE VERSIONS FOR SITTING, STANDING, AMBULATORY
7. RETAIN ESSENCE OF ORIGINAL DANCE

Example of a Dance Adapted for Elderly Groups

The following are three versions of a folk dance activity suitable for different groups. It is based on the traditional "family waltz". There are many varieties of waltzing, swinging and balancing movements which can be performed to gentle or spirited 3/4 music such as: "The Merry Widow Waltz" - Strauss Collection, Columbia Records M34125; "The Anniversary Waltz" - Educational Activities AR85; "Let Me Call You Sweetheart" - Educational Activities AR102, or others like "The Band Played On", "Sunrise, Sunset", "East Side, West Side", "Mexican Waltz", "The Missouri Waltz", and "Beautiful Ohio".

A. Ambulatory - Couple Mixer Version for Active Groups

Dancers stand holding hands in a circle formation facing the center. Partners are designated alternately as "A" or "B".

MEASURES:

1 - 4 four slow rocking movements with one foot in front of the other, toward and away from the center of the circle.

5 - 8 dancers "B" walk four steps in front of "A" to cross over to the other side of partner as dancers "A" take four steps in place.

9-32	repeat measures 1 through 4 three times so that "B" dancers have progressed counterclockwise around the circle to change partners four times altogether.
33	"B" dancers turn to their L, take both hands of "A" facing them
34	partners A & B balance or rock toward each other
35	partners A & B balance or rock away from each other

Ambulatory - Couple Mixer Version for Active Groups (continued)

36	everyone claps their own hands once
37	partners again hold hands and balance toward each other
38	partners balance away from each other
39	partners balance toward each other
40	"A" reaches hands around partners waist, "B" reaches around partners neck and both clap hands in this hugging position
41-46	waltz with partner around room in ballroom dance or two hand hold position
47-48	return to circle with "B" to the right of "A"

Repeat dance from the beginning so that there can be many partner exchanges.

B. Sitting - Partner/Scarf Version for Restricted, Non-Ambulatory Groups

Partners sit facing each other with each one holding an end of the same scarf.

MEASURES:

1-4	dancers "A" in their wheelchairs are pushed slowly toward the center of the circle by aides while dancers "B" are pulled slowly away from the center by aides
5-8	dancers "A" are pulled slowly away from center, while dancers "B" are pushed slowly toward the center
9-16	repeat measures 1 through 8
17-24	dancers are pushed counterclockwise around in a single circle

25-28	aides hold one hand of wheelchair dancers and walk around four steps to end facing them
29-32	partners now hold hands and sway side to side four times
33-36	both partners move their torsos toward each other, away from each other and the aide reaches around to hug seated dancer while clapping behind dancers back
37-44	repeat measures 29 through 36
45-48	aides walk around seated dancers while holding one hand and finish standing in back of wheelchair as at beginning

Dance may be repeated from beginning.

Conclusion

The benefits that can be derived by the elderly who participate in social and popular dancing more than justify the efforts expended to make them appropriate. This valuable source of ethnic and historical material is available to enrich recreational and therapeutic programs for the aging. Leaders who use these vital movement experiences will help validate a cultural heritage. Through the common idioms of these time tested patterns an individual can achieve the sense of relaxation, purpose, and renewal. The dance professional will be able to provide meaningful opportunities for social interaction, physical activity, and personal expression.

REFERENCES

Bartenieff, I. (1972). Dance therapy: A new profession or a rediscovery of an ancient role of dance? Dance Scope, 7, 6-19.

Berger, L.F. & Berger, M.M. (1973). Holistic approach to psychogeriatric outpatient. International Journal Group Psychotherapy, 23, 432-444.

Boxberger, R. & Cotter, V.W. (1968). The geriatric patient. In E.T. Gaston (Ed.), Music in Therapy (pp. 271-280). New York: MacMillan.

Bright, R. (1972). Music in Geriatric Care. New York: St. Martin's Press.

Butler, R.N. (1963). The life review: An interpretation of reminiscence in the aged. Psychiatry, 26, 65-75.

Goldberg, W.G. & Fitzpatrick, J.J. (1980). Movement therapy with the aged. Nursing Research Journal, 29, 339-346.

Hecox, B., Levine, E. & Scott, D. (1976). Dance in physical rehabilitation. Journal Physical Therapy, 58, 919-924.

Helm, J.B. & Gill, K.L. (1974-75). An essential resource for the aging: Dance therapy. Dance Research Journal CORD, 7, (1), 1-7.

Hill, K. (1976). Dance for Physically Handicapped Persons. Reston, VA: American Alliance for Health, Physical Education & Dance.

Layman, E. (1960). Physical activity as a psychiatric adjunct. In W.C. Johnson, (Ed.), Science and Medicine of Exercise and Sports, 623-638. New York: Harper & Row.

Lemon, B., et al. (1972). An explanation of the activity theory of aging: Activity types and life satisfaction among in-movers to a retirement community. Journal of Gerontology, 27, 511-523.

Lindner, E.C., Harpaz, L. & Samberg, S. (1979). Therapeutic Dance/Movement: Expressive Activities for Older Adults. New York: Human Sciences Press.

Lindner, E.C., Harpaz, L. & Samberg, S. . (1977). Special Music for Special People. (AR85). Baldwin, NY: Educational Activities.

Lindner, E.C. & Harpaz, L. (1983). Special Dancing On Your Feet or In Your Seat. (AR102). Baldwin, NY: Educational Activities.

Lindner, E.C. & Harpaz, L. . (1987). Come Dance Again On Your Feet or In Your Seat. (AR103). Baldwin, NY: Educational Activities.

Merritt, M.C. (1971). Dance Therapy Programs in Nursing Homes. Boston, MA: Unitarian Universalist Association.

Rosen, E. (1974). Dance in Psychotherapy. New York: Dance Horizons Publications.

Samuels, A. (1973). Dance therapy for geriatric patients. In Dance Therapist in Dimension: Depth & Diversity, Proceedings of the 8th Annual Conference. (pp. 27-30). Columbia, MD: American Dance Therapy Association.

Sandel, S. (1970). Reminiscence in movement therapy with the aged. Art Psychotherapy, 5, 217-221.

Schoenfeld, L.R. (1977). Psychomotor approach in the nursing home. Dance Magazine, 10, 20-26.

9

Jamaica Dance Forms

Source Of Physical Well-Being For The Older Adult

Sheila Barnett

In the Jamaican society, older adults are active performers in traditional dances such as Ettu, Revival, Bruckins, and the Quadrilles. Endurance, strength, vitality, and skill are linked to knowledge of history, ancestral origins, and religious practices. These older men and women, grandfathers and grandmothers, have preserved their dance heritage and ensured its continuity. Many dance leaders are also prominent citizens, influential in their communities. Teachers to younger generations, they have been active participants and have facilitated the study of the evolution of our dances.

The traditional dance forms permeate and contribute to aspects of the Jamaican lifestyle, while also contributing to the well-being of the people. These dances reflect the dominant African and European (mainly British) influences in the society. Not only are they an integral part of religious expression and secular celebration, but they also reinforce historical perspectives and cultural values. Dancers and spectators are involved. The spectators sing or clap, move to the rhythms, shawl a good dancer, or follow a procession. Jamaicans dance, sing, or play ring games at wakes and fairs. The dance is an instrument of fitness--physical, social and mental--that gives meaning to life.

Physical well-being includes poise which depends as much upon self-worth and self-esteem as it does on muscle strength, endurance, joint freedom, and flexibility. Physicality is influenced by the quality of sensitivity and perception as much as it relies upon the mastery of the body. Good feelings and meaning radiate from the physical interior to beautify the visible exterior.

What do the traditional dances offer as means to improve physical well-being? Through movement, music and meaning, they provide a holistic experience, communicative and non-verbal, that yields individual benefits, stimulates group dynamics, inspires creativity and facilitates social interaction.

Jamaican traditional dances can be categorized as follows:

(A) Dances of African Origin - Kumina and Tambu
(B) Dances of European Origin - Quadrille, Lancers, Maypole
(C) Creolised Dance Forms - Revival Genre - Pocomania and Zion
(D) Urban Folk Forms - Ska, Rocksteady, Raggae, Rasta

The movement vocabulary contained in the traditional dances is rich and varied. It includes:

- Gestures - both occupational and social, through facial expressions and arm and leg movements
- Mime
- Axial movements and the 'playing' of body parts
- Steps and low centered turns, showing the influence of Africa and Europe
- Shuffles and stamps
- Holds and partnering

The style of moving- African influence strongly dictated by:

- Low center of gravity
- Use of flat feet
- Undulating hips
- Flexible ripples and waves of the back
- Twists
- Contractions and releases of the pelvis
- The play between tension and relaxation
- Changes of level
- Directional changes
- Rib cage shifts, thrusts and rotation
- The flat back
- The slow sustained gait
- Wide stance
- Bent knees

The music of the traditional dances of Jamaica include, European chamber and church music that is often laced with polyrhythms and the pulsating beats of Africa. The instruments used are many and varied, either store-bought or improvised. Fife, drum orchestration, percussive instruments, and chants and sounds are used to underscore the meaning of the dance and create the mood. Tempo is varied from slow and easy to fast and exhilarating. Various instruments provide motivation and control the dance execution: cymballing, trumping, tambourine and drum of the revival ceremony complex; mento bands consisting of merimba box (a local relative of the African thumb piano) shackles, craters, guitar and banjo; hand made bamboo instruments like the benta of St. Mary and the stomping tube of St. Elizabeth; and the bass guitar, lead guitar, trap horn and keyboard from reggae.

Meaning is linked to body images, symbols and icons and their influence on the individual. It runs like a vein through the broad cultural base that links movements, structures, religion, community, customs and beliefs. Predominant forms are the circle, longway and square sets, and the columns (of people) that are part of religious and secular processions.

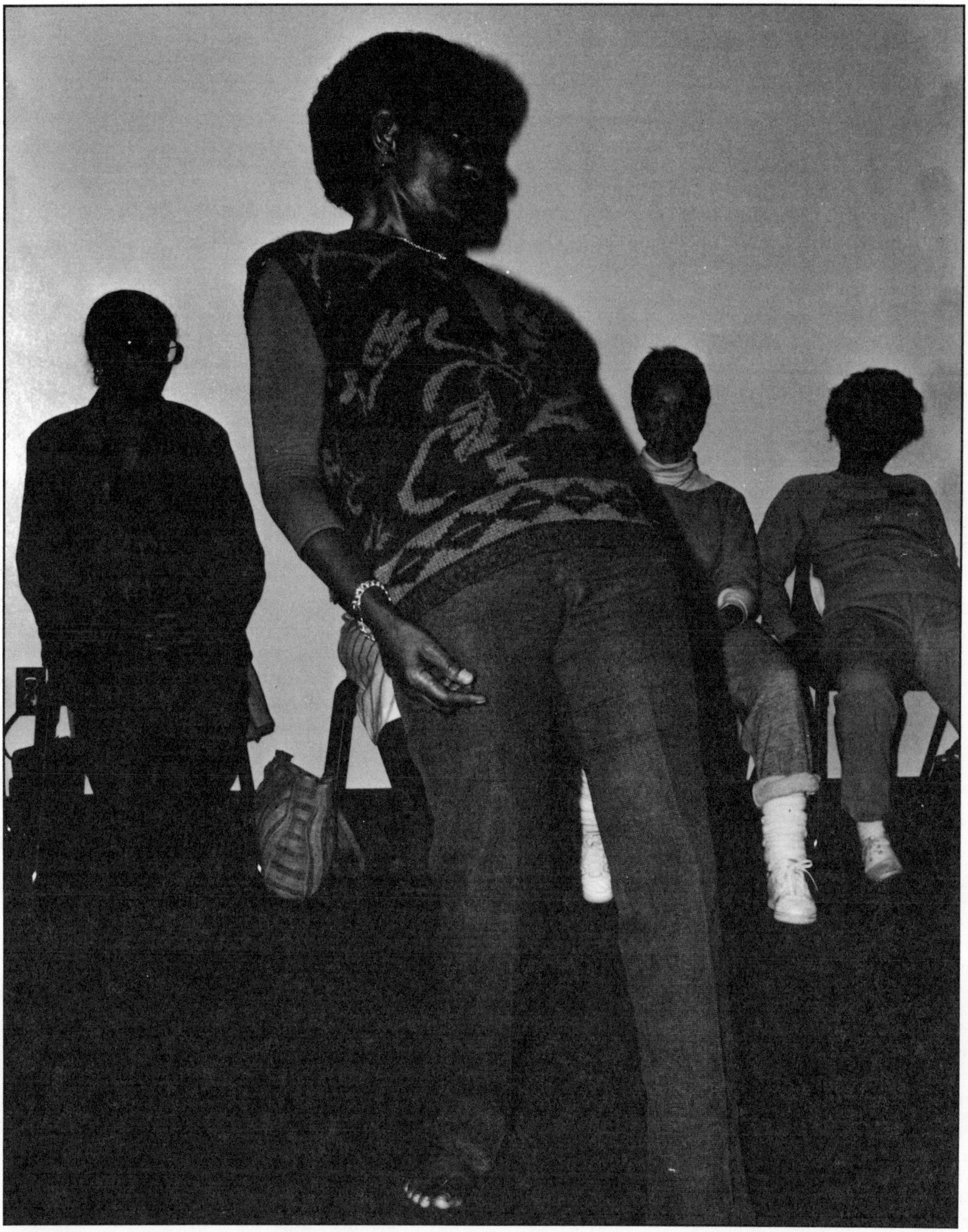

PHOTO COURTESY OF ANDRE RICHARDSON

The traditional dance forms permeate and contribute to aspects of the Jamaican lifestyle while also contributing to the well-being of the people.

Considerations. Use of the traditional Jamaican dance forms to enhance the physical well-being of the older adult to whom these dances are unfamiliar, requires special adaptations and selectivity. Postures and movements must match levels of physical performance. Adjustments, adaptations and the special interest and preferences of the group should be considered. All goals should be attainable. Simple beginnings facilitate better results. Postures and movements may be adapted to levels of physical performance and activities arranged to give enjoyment and a sense of achievement.

Ring-games and integrated songs and dances are good starters. The vocabulary and pattern content of both the ring-games and integrated song and dance prepare the dancers for further involvement. Teaching approaches using dramatic and/or competitive situations linked to specific traditional dances, together with background information about the dances, develop interest and increase learning readiness.

The vocabulary and content of Jamaican traditional dances can provide sufficient material for a program by balancing aesthetics and physical activities aimed at creating a more vital life style. Because these dances are rooted in human experience and life issues, they can give new insights, perceptions and an understanding of others. The traditional material is a movement source for further manipulation.

Creativity is vital to a satisfying life-style at any age. A person who can think and act creatively reassesses his worth. Movement experiences, both new and remembered, provide the older adult with social interaction, physical vitality, and a renewed sense of self-esteem. "To dance is to live," states Professor Opoku of the University of Ghana, really means "to dance is to maintain life."

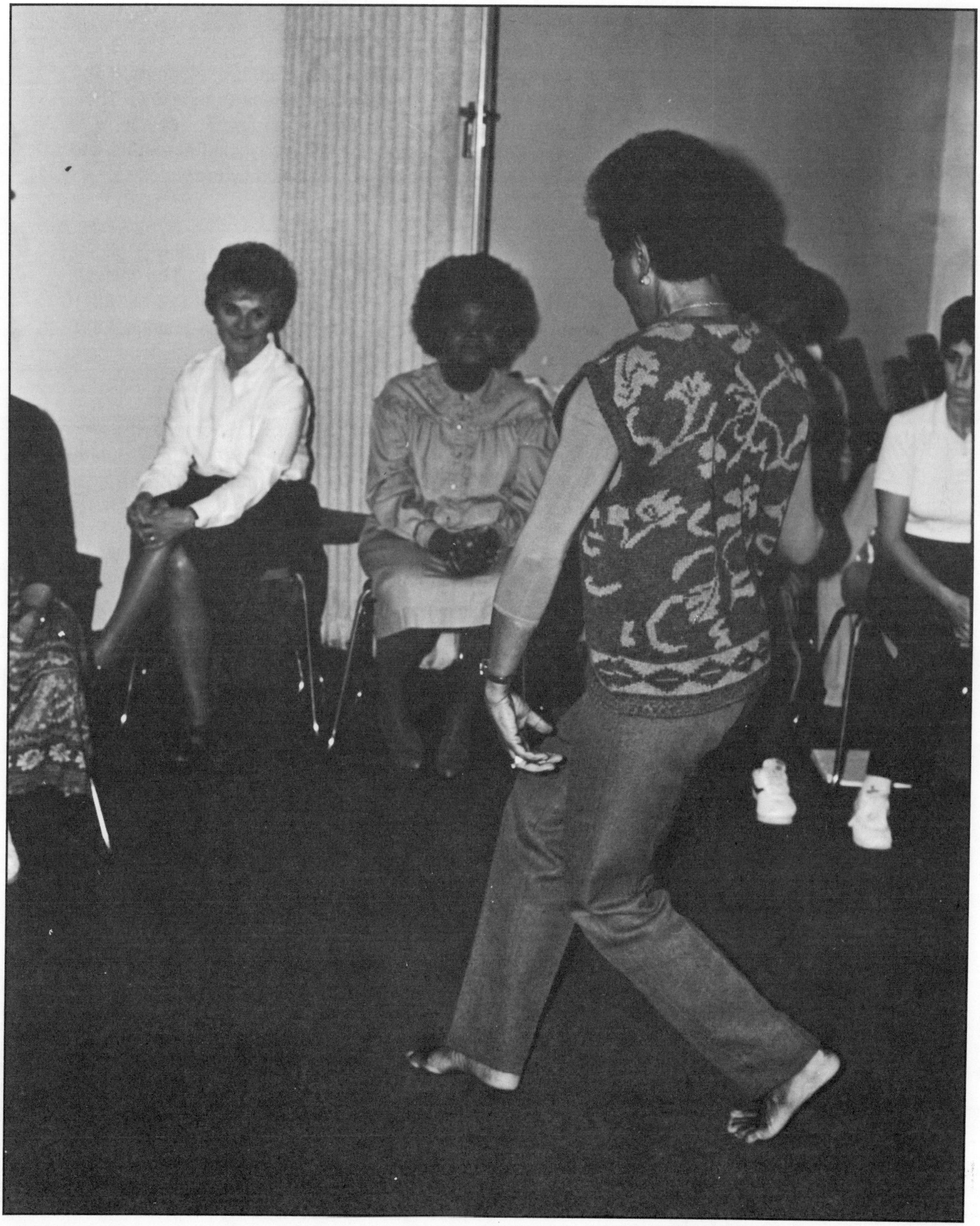

PHOTO COURTESY OF ANDRE RICHARDSON

Bruckins Party **is a creolised dance form uniting the British and African influences.**

DANCE DESCRIPTION

1. ETTU	- African retention found in the Parish of Hanover. The dancers claim to be of Yoruba (Nigerian) ancestry. The food of the Ettu feast is African in origin. The dance is performed on many occasions which include funerals and weddings. Good dancers are shawled by the 'Queen' or a lead dancer.
2. REVIVAL	- Includes Pukkumina and Zion Afro-Christian Religions. Dancing is part of the religious expression. The revival band arose out of the religious movement (1880-1881) called the great revival. Symbolism, role-playing, and possession are important features of this religious complex.
3. BRUCKINS PARTY	- Is found mainly in the parish of St. Thomas. It is a creolised dance form uniting the British and African influences. Originally this dance was performed as part of the anniversary celebrations of emancipation (1838). Today Bruckins is danced on many social occasions. Each group has a queen and two sets of dancers dressed in red or blue. Each set strives to outdance the other.
4. QUADRILLE	- The Quadrille was brought to Jamaica from Europe by the British. It flourished in the 19th century. Two types of Quadrille are performed: the stately ballroom and the informal country. The forms remain European but styles have been influenced by the drum sound and African nuances.
5. CYMBALLING	- The shrill singing that accompanies the revival ritual. The lead voice cuts across the trumping beat carried by the worshippers.
6. TRUMPING	- Forms the pulse across which cymballing cuts. It could be described as a grunt made at regular intervals that is done with a forceful expulsion of breath and obvious use of the chest - overbreathing.

7. MENTO - This is a social dance/music form that was very popular in the 40's and 50's and early 60's. It combines influences that are African/traditional, Cuban Rhumba, and European.

8. BENTA - Found in the Parish of St. Mary. A bamboo length of 4' to 5' is placed horizontally on two supports. The skin on one side of the bamboo is raised in straight strips to form the strings which are supported on small wooden lifts. It is played by two musicians, one sitting at each end. One musician rubs a large hollowed gourd back and forth along the strings. The other uses two sticks to make rhythmic sounds. The resulting music along with the drums have a hypnotic effect. The music and dance are used at wakes.

9. STOMPING TUBE - Found in the Parish of St. Elizabeth, this dance uses a bamboo tube about 5 feet long. It is held upright near the top and is used to strike the ground.

REFERENCES

Author Unknown (1976). Ettu people of Hanover. Peenie Wallie, 1, (2), pp.13-16.

Barnett, S., The root of the matter: Hybridism and caribbean dance theatre. Proceedings of the 8th Commonwealth International Conference, Glasgow Scotland, 1986.

Campbell, D.J. (1976) Jamaican folk and traditional dance. Jamaica Journal, 10, (1), pp. 8-9.

Hawkins, A. (1965) Creating Through Dance. Englewood Cliffs, NJ: Prentice-Hall Inc.

Ryman, C. (1984) African Retentions in Jamaican Traditional Dance. Inside Jamaica, 3, (1), pp. 18-21.

III. Research

10

The Aging Process

Benefits of Physical Activity

Everett L. Smith And Sally K. Zook

All living creatures age. Aging is species-specific and controlled by the genetic makeup of the cell. Aging can be defined chronologically or physiologically. Physiological aging is the loss of the ability to adapt to one's environment. Peak physiological function is reached at approximately age 30, after which, in sedentary persons, physiological capabilities decline. Functional declines are evident in work capacity, cardiac output, heart rate, blood pressure, respiration, basal metabolic rate, musculature, nerve conduction, flexibility, bone, and total body water (see Table 1). To curtail the effects of aging, an adaptive physical training program allowing individuals to maintain peak function for their age is desirable. Physical activity programs for older adults must be based on the physiological capabilities and limitations of the participants.

Functional physiological decline

Biological functional decline with age is a complex process, with variation both within and between individuals. While the average decline of various systems can be given, it must be kept in mind that not all individuals demonstrate the same characteristics. The rate of change depends on the individual's lifestyle and heritage. It is difficult to delineate which declines are specifically age related because of the interaction of aging per se with disuse atrophy or disease. The following text summarizes physiological and anatomical changes with age in the sedentary U.S. population and the effects of physical activity on the aging process.

Basal metabolic rate

The average 70-year-old has a lower resting metabolic rate and a lower energy expenditure per day. As a result, weight and fat increase while muscle mass declines. Tzankoff and Norris (1977) indicated that the decline in basal metabolic rate is directly related to the decline in muscle mass. Changes in body composition and in sweating mechanisms result in less heat tolerance in older adults. Reduced total body water makes older adults more susceptible to dehydration, and greater body fat accompanied by a delayed onset of sweating make them more susceptible to heat stroke. Older adults participating in a physical activity program should be aware of the necessity of remaining hydrated and of avoiding excessively hot environments.

Neuromuscular

Age-related decreases in muscle mass are well documented, with the quadriceps muscle suffering the earliest and greatest decline. Skeletal muscle consists of both slow and fast twitch fibers. With age, fast twitch muscle fiber decreases more rapidly than slow twitch. The overall loss of muscle mass and greater loss of fast twitch fiber compromise strength and endurance in older adults.

Research on the effects of physical activity on neuromuscular changes in the aging population is sparse, and the conclusions are controversial. McCafferty and Edington (1970) hypothesize that there may be an age beyond which training no longer stimulates muscle hypertrophy in either the skeletal muscle or the heart. However, Petrofsky and Lind (1975) observed no difference in muscular strength or endurance of men between 25 and 65 performing similar work activities in an aircraft corporation machine shop.

Suominen, Heikkinen and Parkatti (1977) studied 69-year-old men and women who completed an eight-week physical activity program held for one hour, five times a week. They concluded that older adults have improvements in fitness and muscle similar to the young.

De Lorme and Watkins (1951) hypothesized a two-stage process for strength gain: increased nerve activity followed by muscle hypertrophy. Moritani (1981) trained both young and old men in an eight-week isotonic strength-training regimen. Young subjects increased both neural activity and muscle mass; older subjects increased neural function only. Further research is necessary to determine if muscle hypertrophy can be induced in the older adult with different training techniques or longer exercise regimes.

Flexibility

Declines in flexibility in the aging population are so consistent that Allman (1974) suggested flexibility as an index of physiological aging. Johns and Wright (1962) reported that connective tissue changes in muscle, ligaments, joint capsules, and tendons were responsible for 98 percent of flexibility loss. The decline of flexibility, however, is more strongly correlated to disuse than to age degeneration.

Few research programs have tested the effects of physical activity on flexibility in older adults. Chapman, deVries, and Swezey (1972) studied joint stiffness in 20 young and 20 old adults. After a six-week training program both groups showed the same amount of improvement. Lesser (1978) studied 60 elderly subjects who exercised for ten weeks and found a significant improvement in flexibility at two-thirds of the sites measured. Munns (1981) worked with 40 elderly subjects, 20 of these serving as controls. After 12 weeks, the exercise group had improved at all sites (neck, shoulder, wrist, knee, hip, and ankle) by eight to 48 percent.

Cardiovascular

The cardiovascular system declines 30 percent between ages 30 and 70 in its ability to deliver blood to the tissues. This decline results from changes in the heart and vascular system. The heart muscle is weaker and maximum heartrate is lower. Blood vessels lose elasticity and become narrow, increasing the resistance to blood flow.

The benefits of physical activity are well documented in the young, but have yet to be adequately demonstrated in the older adult. Few researchers have studied long-term physical activity programs. In one of these few studies, Kasch and Wallace (1976) demonstrated that individuals over 45 participating in an aerobic physical activity program over a 10 to 15-year period did not, on the average, decline in cardiovascular fitness.

Studies of shorter duration have shown improvements in aerobic power and general cardiovascular fitness (Morse & Smith, 1981), declines in resting systolic blood pressure (deVries, 1970), and exercise systolic blood pressure (Stamford, 1972). A study by Sidney and Shephard (1978) reported intensity and frequency to be important factors in producing a training effect. No response was observed in subjects who exercised less than twice a week at heart rates less than 120. From the available research it is apparent that physical activity can enhance the overall physical fitness of older adults, as well as provide increased ease of participation in daily life activities.

Respiratory and sensory

Various studies show that total lung capacity does not decrease with age. However, vital capacity and and residual volume are affected by the aging process.

Changes in lung tissue decreased the availability of oxygen to the cardiovascular system. The lung decreases in the capacity to expire and an increased residual volume. The total surface area of the lung decreases 25 to 30 percent between 30 to 70 years. This, in conjunction with other alterations in the thorax, results in a decreased blood oxygen.

While the lung functions well at rest and during mild exercise, vigorous exercise is limited in the average older adult due to a greater work load of moving a stiffer thorax, increased residual volume, physiological shunting and, thus, decreased levels of blood oxygenation.

All individuals over 60 experience abatement of sensory function to some degree. The neurological and mechanical systems of hearing decline, resulting in decreased auditory acuity and ability to hear high-pitched sounds. Visual acuity, depth perception, and sensitivity to glare are also affected by age.

Bone mineral content

Bone loss presents a significant problem for women over 60 and men over 80. More than six million elderly men and women in the United States have a significant degree of bone loss.

Men over 50 lose about 0.4 percent per year in bone mass. Women, however, lose approximately one to two percent per year from age 35. This loss accelerates to four to five percent per year in the period immediately following menopause. As a result, 60 to 70-year-old women are prone to fractures of the hip, wrist, and spine and to an overall loss of skeletal integrity.

The role of physical activity in the prevention of bone loss with age has yet to be delineated. It is clear that gravity or weight bearing and muscle contraction are necessary for bone maintenance (Donaldson et al., 1970; Krolner and Toft, 1983; Mack, 1967). If either gravity or muscle contraction is significantly reduced or increased, bone formation and removal are affected.

Numerous studies of humans demonstrate that bone hypertrophies with exercise. In athletes, those bones which endure the greatest amounts of mechanical stress demonstrate the greatest hypertrophy (Dalen & Olsson, 1974).

Physical activity can affect bone mineral mass regardless of age. While continued research is needed to delineate the specific activities necessary to prevent bone loss, it appears that physical activity may play a key role in the maintenance of skeletal integrity.

Table 1. Biological functional changes between the ages of 30 and 70.

Biological Function	Change
Work capacity (%)[1]	25-30
Cardiac output (%)[4,5]	30
Maximum heart rate (beats/min^{-1})[6]	24
Blood pressure (mm Hg)[7]	
Systolic	10-40
Diastolic	05-10
Respiration (%)[8-9]	
Vital capacity	40-50
Residual volume	30-50
Basal metabolic rate (%)[10]	08-12
Musculature (%)[11-13]	
Muscle mass	25-30
Hand grip strength	25-30
Nerve conduction velocity (%)[14]	10-15
Flexibility (%)[15]	20-30
Bone (%)[16,17]	
Women	25-30
Men	15-20
Renal function (%)[18]	30-50

Reprinted by permission of The Physician and Sportsmedicine, a McGraw-Hill Publication.

REFERENCES

Allman, F.L. (1974). Conditioning for sports. In A.J. Ryan & F.L. Allman (Eds.), *Sports Medicine.* New York: Academic Press.

Chapman, E.A., deVries, H.A., & Swezey, R. (1972). Joint stiffness: Effects of exercise on young and old men. *Journal of Gerontology,* 27(2), 218-221.

Dalen, N., & Olsson, K.E. (1974). Bone mineral content and physical activity. *Acta Orthopedica Scaninavia,* 45, 170-174.

De Lorme, T.L., & Watkins, A.L. (1951). *Progressive resistance exercise.* New York: Appleton Century, Inc.

deVries, H.A. 91970). Physiological effects of an exercise training regimen upon men aged 52-88. *Journal of Gerontology,* 25, 325-336.

Donaldson, C., Halley, S.B., Vogel, J.M., Hattner, R.S., Bayers, J.H., & MacMillan, D.E., (1970). Effect of prolonged bedrest on bone mineral. *Metabolism,* 19, 12, 1071-1084.

Johns, R.J., & Wright, U. (1962). Relative importance of various tissues in joint stiffness. *Journal of Applied Physiology,* 17, 824-828.

Kasch, F.W., & Wallace, J.P. (1976). Physiological variables during 10 years of endurance exercise. *Medicine and Science in Sports and Exercise,* 8(1), 5-8.

Krolner, b., & Toft, B. (1983). Vertebral bone loss: An unheeded side effect of therapeutic bed rest. *Clinical Science,* 64, 537-540.

Lesser, M. (1978). The effects of rhythmic exercise on the range of motion in older adults. *American Corrective Therapy Journal,* 32(4), 118-122.

Mack, P., LaChance, P., Vose, G., & Vogt, F. (1967). Bone demineralization of foot and hand on Gemini-Titan IV, V, and VII astronauts during orbital flight. *American Journal of Roentgenology,* 100, 503,511.

McCafferty, W.B., & Edington, D.W. (1970). Skeletal muscle and organ weights of aged and trained male rats. *Gerontology,* 20, 44-50.

Moritani, T. (1981). Training adaptations in the muscles of older men. In E.L. Smith & R.C. Serfass (Eds.), *Exercise and aging: The scientific basis.* Hillside, NJ: Enslow Publishers.

Morse, C.E., & Smith, E.L. (1981). Physical activity programming for the aged. In E.L. Smith & R.C. Serfass (Eds.), *Exercise and aging: The scientific basis.* Hillside, NJ: Enslow Publishers.

Munns, K. (1981). Effects of exercise on the range of joint motion. In E.L. Smith & R.C. Serfass (Eds.), *Exercise and aging: The scientific basis.* Hillside, NJ: Enslow Publishers.

Petrofsky, J.S., & Lind, A.R. (1975). Aging, isometric strength and endurance, and cardiovascular responses to static effort. *Journal of Applied Physiology,* 39, 91-95.

Sidney, K.H., & Shephard, R.J. (1978). Frequency and intensity of exercise training for elderly subjects. *Medicine and Science in Sports and Exercise,* 10, 125-131.

Stamford, B.A. (1972). Physiological effects of training upon institutionalized geriatric men. *Journal of Gerontology*, 27(4), 451-455.

Suominen, H., Heikkinen, E., & Parkatti, T. (1977). Effect of eight weeks physical training on muscle and conductive tissue of the M. vastus lateralis in 69-year-old men and women. *Journal of Gerontology*, 32(1), 33-37.

Tzankoff, S.P., & Norris, A.H. (1977). Effect of muscle mass decrease on age-related BMR changes. *Journal of Applied Physiology*, 43(6), 1001-1006.

11

A Dance Activities Program For The Older Adult

Rayma K. Beal

The life expectancy for the average American is steadily increasing. For example, in 1900 the number of people over the age of 65 comprised 4.1 percent of the population. In 1970 there were 20,177,000 people over the age of 65, comprising 9.9 percent of the population. Currently there are about 41 million people in that age group comprising 20 percent of the population. It is estimated that this figure will climb to 59 million people by the year 2000 and comprise 25 percent of the population. This increase in life expectancy appears to be the result of better medical care, better living conditions, better diet and nutrition (Cutler and Harootyan, 1975).

Unfortunately, this increased life expectancy is accompanied by numerous problems, and the negative consequences of old age can include social isolation and depression. Indeed, depression is the most frequent psychological complaint of the older adult (Perlin and Butler, 1963; Busse, 1970). Other emotional problems facing the older adult are increased anxiety, and severe decreases in life satisfaction (Harris, 1975). Additionally, there are a number of physical consequences which accompany old age, the most notable being a reduction in physical activity, reduced heart rate, and reduced blood flow.

In order to address these serious psychological and physical complaints, a number of researchers have begun to examine the effects of exercise programs for decreasing depression, decreasing anxiety, and increasing life satisfaction. For example, Bennett, Carmack, and Gardner (1982) studied the effects of regular physical exercise on levels of depression in older adults. These researchers found that there was a significant decrease in depression, and a significant increase in the subject's physical functioning following an eight-week physical exercise program. Adams and deVries (1973) studied the effect of a twelve-week exercise program involving calisthentics, jogging, and stretching on a group of women between the ages of 52 and 79 years. These researchers found a significant improvement in resting heart rate capacity at the end of the training program. Holder (1983) found participation in an eight-week aerobic exercise program produces statistically significant decreases in depression level, and significant decrements in diastolic blood pressure among the elderly, when compared to a non-treatment group. Finally, Reiter (1981), studied the effects of exercise on selected mood states, such as anxiety, tension, depression and general well being. Reiter found significant reductions in state anxiety, and improvement in feelings of well being, following the completion of an exercise program. Specifically, Reiter's experimental group felt more relaxed, less tense and anxious, and they reported feeling more awake and vital during the day, and better able to sleep at night. The control group did not evidence _any_ of these changes. Thus, it appears that exercise programs with older adults improve both physiological functioning and psychological functioning as well. Specifically, exercises that maximize rhythmic activity of large muscle groups appear to decrease anxiety and depression, and improve feelings of life satisfaction.

A second body of empirical research having strong implications for dance professionals focuses on increasing social support among the elderly. That is, increased social behavior appears to be strongly correlated with physical well being (Berkman and Syme, 1979; Blazer, 1982). A frequently cited study relating health and social support is a nine year follow-up of residents of Alameda County (Berkman and Syme, 1979). These researchers found that persons with fewer social ties suffered mortality rates an average of 2.6 times higher that those persons who reported greater social support. Furthermore, (Blazer, 1982) obtained similar findings. That is, Blazer found mortality rates 3.5 times higher for persons who perceived lower levels of social support that their socially supported counterparts. Miller and Ingham (1976) found that persons claiming to have "few acquaintances" had the most negative physical symptoms, whereas persons having "some acquaintances" had significantly fewer symptoms. In short, there appears to be a growing body of evidence suggesting that individuals derive strong positive benefits from social interaction and social support.

It would appear that these two bodies of research (the body of research suggesting that physical exercise significantly decreases depression and anxiety and the body of research suggesting that individuals derive physical and psychological benefits from social interaction) are particularly relevant to dance professionals, in that dance activities, in there many forms, can become a satisfying element in any exercise program (Adkins, 1981). Indeed, social, folk, ballet, modern, and jazz dance have movement qualities that are helpful in developing and maintaining flexibility, strength, range of motion, and rhythm. Further, dance programs are easily structured to enhance social support.

The present paper attempts to demonstrate that a dance activities program can provide major benefits of a physical exercise program, and additionally, can develop a strong social support network among its members. Furthermore, it is suggested that a dance-activities program circumvents the most common criticism of most exercise programs, namely that "exercise is boring" by varying the dance activities. Finally, it was thought that such a study would provide a valuable contribution to the literature, in that it would combine both the positive advantages of an exercise program with the positive benefits of a group program which was established to increase social interaction.

Subjects

Twenty-five active/independent older adults, selected from a population of volunteers who frequented a senior citizens center, made up the subject population. These active/independent older adults were individuals between the ages of 60 and 80, who were _not_ confined to a nursing home or institution, but rather individuals who lived in their own home in the community, and frequented a community center for senior citizens. None of these individuals showed signs of severe withdrawal associated with paranoia, schizophrenia, or severe senile dementia. These individuals were ambulatory, although some needed assistance with physical activities due to injury or arthritis in the foot, knee, shoulder, or other parts of the body. Some of these individuals experienced mild hearing loss or visual impairment, but over-all, their general health was fair to good. The population was primarily female, who were predominantly white, and of middle socio-economic class. Subject characteristics were as follows: the mean age of the control group was 68.84 years. There was no significant difference between the groups in terms of age, t (23) = 1.52, p>.05.

With respect to marital status, the modal status was widowed, with 50 percent of both the experimental and control groups being widowed. The distribution by marital status is shown in Table I. The racial composition of the group was predominantly white (88 percent). There was one black subject in the experimental group, and two black subjects in the control group. The other 22 subjects in the study were white. The subjects in the study were all women, except for one man in the control group.

TABLE I

Means and Standard Deviations on Relevant Demographic Characteristics for the Dance/Activities and Control Groups

CHARACTERISTICS	DANCE/ACTIVITIES	CONTROL
N	12	13
Age		
M	72.6	68.8
SD	6.49	6.06
Marital Status		
Married	2	5
Widowed	6	6
Divorced	2	0
Single	2	2
Sex		
Female	12	12
Male	0	1
Race		
White	11	11
Black	1	2

Dependent Measures

One of the primary characteristics of the geriatric patients is increased depression, increased anxiety, and decreased life satisfaction (Perlin and Butler, 1963; Busse, 1970; Harris, 1975). Therefore, it was expected that the dance activities program, presented over an extended period of time would significantly decrease depression, significantly decrease anxiety, and significantly improve life satisfaction.

To assess the degree of depression, the Beck Depression Inventory (BDI) was selected as the measure of choice because it is one of the most widely used, and thoroughly validated self-report measures of depression. The stability criteria and internal consistency obtained from a large out-patient psychiatric population (N= 606) resulted in a Pearson rating of .93 (Beck, 1967). Additionally, computation of the correlation between the BDI and clinicians rating for various samples, including a general medical sample by Beck and his colleagues (1974), found that the BDI correlated .67 with physicians ratings of depression.

The possible range of scores obtainable of the BDI is 0-63 points. A score of 1-10 points indicates the normal ups and downs of mood shifts. Scores between 11 and 16 indicate mild mood disturbance. Scores between 17 and 20 indicate borderline clinical depression. Scores between 21 and 30 indicate moderate depression. Scores between 31 and 40 indicate severe depression, and a score over 40 is an indication of extreme depression. A score of 17 or above indicates the need for professional treatment (Beck, 1967).

The second dependent measure used in present study was the Life Satisfaction Index (LSI). The LSI assumes that Life Satisfaction is a multi-dimensional concept (Knapp, 1976). The LSI is a 20 item scale, measuring the extent to which respondent: (1) takes pleasure from the types of activities that constitute his every day life, (2) regards his life as meaningful and accepts resolutely that which has been, (3) feels he has succeeded in achieving his major goals, (4) follows a positive self-image, and (5) maintains a happy and optimistic attitude and mood (Neugarten, Havinghurst, and Tobin, 1961). The LSI is a 20-item questionnaire, with a three-choice answer scale. Scores on the LSI range from 0 to 20.

The LSI is a measure of psychological well being that is relatively independent of the level of activity or social participation of the respondents, and is familiar to most Gerontologists. This index relies on the respondents internal frame of reference rather than his overt behavior, and solicits information concerning a subject's feelings of happiness and satisfaction with life (Harris, 1975).

Finally, this study is directly concerned with the observation that as people age, they tend to socially withdraw. As noted above, this social withdrawal tends to exacerbate their situation, and result in significantly higher mortality rates, as well as resulting in increased depression, anxiety, and a sense of isolation. Thus, any sort of intervention which increases verbal interaction, may well reduce this tendency towards isolation. As such, the assessment verbal interaction was chosen as a dependent measure. Verbal interaction was defined using the criteria of Matarazzo and Weins (1972). A verbalization unit consists of verbal units that are separated at either end by a silence -- one silence following another participants last comment, and the other silence followed by the speakers own comment and preceding another participant's comment. The utterance included all pauses that were suggested by the content to be part of the expression of the same idea or thought. However, when pauses preceded the introduction of a whole new idea or thought by the speaker himself, this signaled the introduction of a second speech unit.

In each of the measurement periods, the verbal interaction was recorded by the researcher. The actual dependent measures were obtained at the first and final meetings, schedules at a definite time, for which the researcher was deliberately ten minutes late. During this delay, the verbal interactions and responses of the group members were observed without the group members awareness of the recording by the researcher. This measure was of particular interest, since it more closely resembled common social encounters in daily living.

Procedure

The subjects were randomly assigned to one of two treatment conditions. The two groups were then pre-tested. Subsequently, the experimental group received 16 sessions of dance/activities therapy, during an eight week period, while the control group was a waiting list control. That is, the control subjects were allowed to complete pre-test measures, but were told that they would be placed on a waiting list, and their group would begin in eight weeks. After the initial eight week phase was concluded, each group was post-tested. Following the completion of the experimental phase, the waiting list control group began its dance activities program.

Treatment

Each treatment session began with the members taking their pulse. This was done by their sitting quietly in a chair and taking their pulse either from the radial artery or the carotid artery. The class then began selected dance movements consisting of sitting, stretching exercises and warm-ups, for approximately five minutes. The group then progressed to torso movements involving the hands, arms, chest, and neck. The movement then progressed to the lower body. Following a thorough warm-up period, the experimental group proceeded through a dance activity, consisting of various dances over time. For example, basic social dance steps were used, as were folk dances, the Hula, and Charleston. Dance activities selected for this program were based on the work by Caplow-Lindner, Harpaz and Samberg (1979), Corbin and Metal-Corbin (1983), Adkins (1981), Lerman (1984) and Rosenberg (1977). In addition, basic techniques in modern dance, jazz, and ballet were used. (A complete description of dance activities and musical accompaniment appropriate for older adults is available from the author.)

At the end of the dance activities session, each group member took and recorded their pulse rate a second time. At the beginning of the final session, the examiner was deliberately ten minutes late, in order that a measure of verbal interaction could be completed. Then, each participant also completed a second BDI, and a second Life Satisfaction Inventory.

For the control group, they merely completed the verbal interaction task, the BDI, and the Life Satisfaction Inventory at a first meeting, and then at a meeting approximately eight weeks later.

It might be noted that the community center where the dance activities program took place had weekly pot luck luncheons where once-a-month birthdays and anniversaries were celebrated. At this meeting, entertainment often included members of the dance group, performing dances they learned in the program. For example, at one of the monthly meetings, the dance activities group performed a Hula, and at another the Charleston. These activities provided the members with the opportunity to experience the performance component of dancing as well as to receive positive social support from their peers.

Results

Statistical analysis of the results of the Beck Depression Inventory and the Life Satisfaction Index resulted in no statistically significant differences between groups. That is, the procedure did not

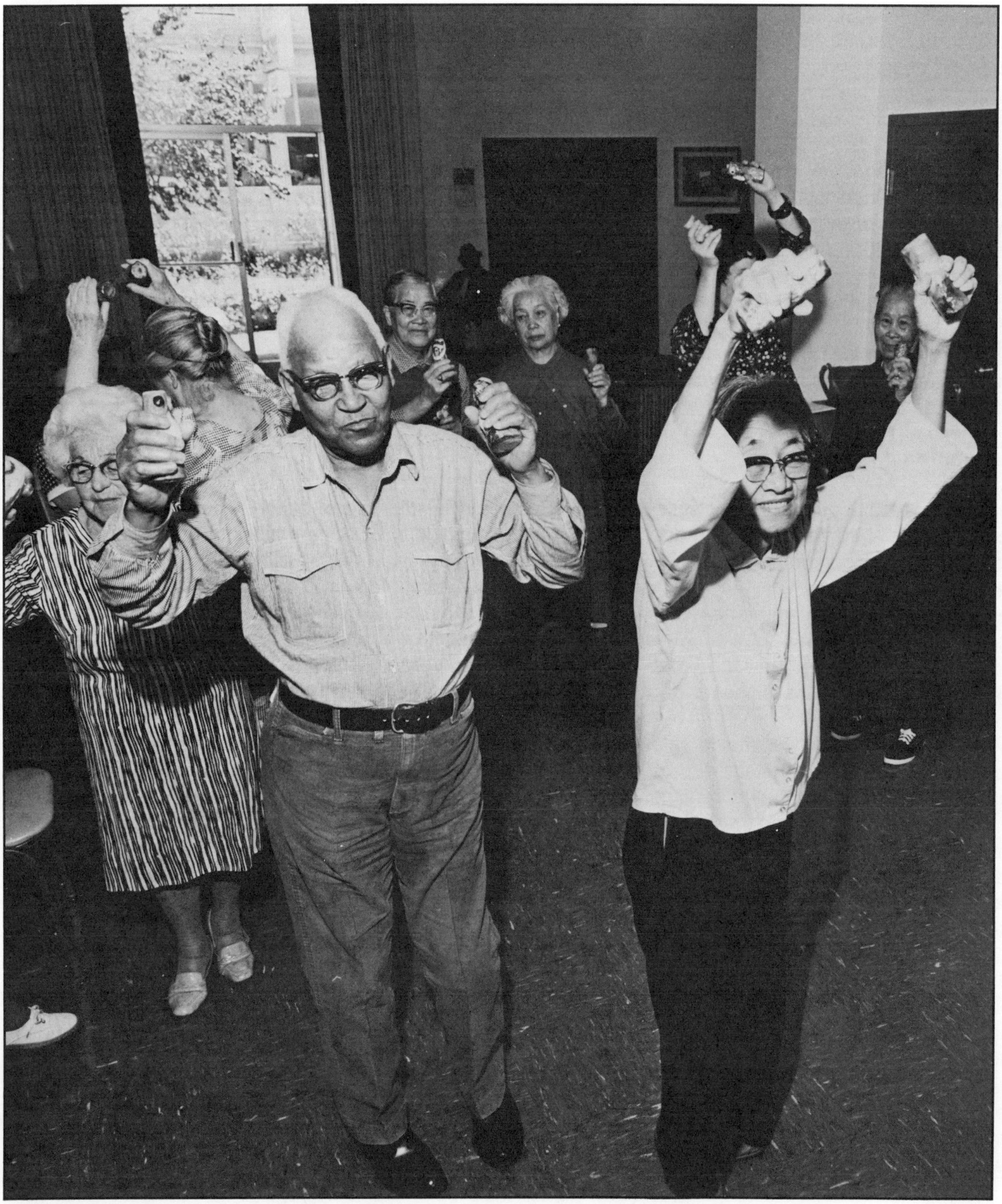

A dance activity program can help in significantly reducing social isolation in active, older adults.

appear to be effective in reducing subjective depression, or increasing life satisfaction as measured by the BDI and the LSI. These non-significant results on the BDI and the LSI appear to be the result of the fact that the average BDI score and LSI score fell well within the range of "normal ups and downs". Also increased depression, and decreased life satisfaction appears to be correlates of individuals living in nursing homes. In the present case, these individuals were living in the community, were fairly active in the community, and both their pre- and post-test results fell in the "normal ups and down range".

With respect to the data on social interaction, prior to the analysis of the dependent measures, the data were examined for adherence to the assumptions of analysis of variance techniques. The data was positively skewed and did not meet the homogeneity of variance assumption. Therefore, the Mann Whitney procedure was utilized (Kirk, 1968). This statistical technique, (based on the median) is not affected by the extreme responsiveness of only one or two members. Thus, the statistical differences do fairly reflect actual group differences in level of interaction.

An analysis of the pre-test scores in the verbal interaction tasks showed no differences among groups. Post test medians, however, were significantly different, U (n 1=13, n 2=12) = 10, $p < .01$. With the dance activities group demonstrating significantly more verbal action than the control group

Discussion

The results of the present study offer strong support for the use of dance activities group in increasing social interaction among active/independent older adults. On the other hand, there did not seem to be significant improvement in life satisfaction, or a significant decrease in depression. This however, is not surprising. The treatment groups life satisfaction scores, and their depression scores were well within the normal range. Indeed, their scores fell within the range that would be considered the "daily ups and downs" of life. Nevertheless, in the context of a controlled experiment using objectively defined behavioral measures, the dance activities program was clearly effective in increasing verbal interaction among members of a group that is frequently socially isolated in the community.

Another point which should be emphasized concerns gains accrued by the experimental group members, which were not measured by the Beck Depression Inventory or the Life Satisfaction Scale. That is, feedback from the verbal responses of subject themselves, as well as feedback from the Director of the Community Center, suggested that the treatment program had a significant impact on the participants in areas other than life satisfaction and depression. The activities seemed to provide noticeable social interaction for participants and in this way was a meaningful activity to participate in. In addition, the dance activity program attracted additional members to the Senior Citizens Group. Thus, the program appears to address one of the other serious problems of aging, mainly social isolation.

In summary, the present study offers cause for optimism regarding the benefits of a dance activities program for older adults. In general, the findings suggests that a dance activities program helps in significantly reducing social isolation in active independent older adults. While the study did not seem to affect anxiety, depression, or life satisfaction, it is argued that this study was not an adequate test of that hypothesis, in that individuals who experienced increased depression, and decreased life satisfaction are largely individuals confined to rest homes. It is hypothesized that in the nursing home setting, one would likely observe decreased depression, increased life satisfaction, as well as increased social interaction.

REFERENCES

Adams, G.M. and deVries, H.A. (1973). Physiological effects of an exercise training regime upon women ages 52-79. Journal of Gerontology, 28, 50-55.

Adkins, O.B. (1981). Get moving! Exercise for later life. Oxford, OH: Scripps Foundation Gerontology Center.

Beck, A.T. (1967). Depression: Causes and treatments. Philadelphia: University of Pennsylvania Press.

Beck, A.T. (1974). Depressive neurosis. In S. Arieti (Ed.). American handbook of psychiatry (2nd ed.) New York: Basic Books.

Bennett, J., Carmack, M.A., and Gardner, V.J. (1982). The effects of a program of physical exercise on depression in older adults. Physical Educator, 39 (1), 21-24.

Berkman, L., and Syme, S.L. (1979). Social networks, host resistance and mortality. A nine year follow-up of Alameda County residents. American Journal of Epidemiology, 109. 186-204.

Blazer, D.G. (1982). Social support and mortality in an elderly community population. American Journal of Epidemiology, 115, 684-694.

Busse, E. (1970). Psychoneurotic reactions and defense mechanisms in the aged. In E. Palmon (Ed.). Normal aging: Reports from the Duke longitudinal study. Durham, NC: Duke University Press.

Caplow-Lindner, E., Harpaz, L., and Samberg, S. (1979). Therapeutic dance/movement: Expressive activities for older adults. New York: Human Sciences Press.

Corbin, D.E. and Metal-Corbin, J. (1983). Reach for it: A handbook of exercise and dance activities for older adults. Dubuque, IA: Eddie Bowers.

Cutler, N.E. and Harootyan, R.A. (1975). Demography of the aged. In D.S. Woodruff and J.E. Birren (Eds.). Aging: Scientific perspectives and social issues. New York: D. Van Nostrand.

Harris, J.E. (1975). The effect of activity therapy as a treatment for disengaged community-residing elderly persons. (Doctoral dissertation, Texas Tech University, 1975). University Microfilms No. 75-26, 842.

Holder, J.D. (1983). The effect of low level aerobic activity upon systolic blood pressure, heart rate, and depression levels among the elderly. (Doctoral dissertation, Boston University School of Education.) Dissertation Abstracts International, 43, 3817 A.

Kirk, R. (1968). Experimental design procedures for the behavioral sciences. Monterrey, CA: Brooks Cole.

Knapp, M.R.J. (1976). Predicting the dimensions of life satisfaction. Journal of Gerontology, 31, 594-604.

Lerman, L. (1984). Teaching dance to senior adults. Springfield, IL: Charles C. Thomas.

Matarazzo, J. and Wiens, A. (1972). *The interview: Research on its anatomy and structure.* Chicago: Aldine, 1972

Miller, P. and Ingham, J.G. (1976). Friends, confidants and symptoms. *Social Psychiatry, 11,* 51-58.

Neugarten, B.L., Havinghurst, R.J., and Tobin, S.S. (1961). The measurement of life satisfaction. *Journal of Gerontology, 16,* 134-143.

Perlin, S. and Butler, R.N. (1963). Psychiatric aspects of adaptation to the aging experience. In J.E. Birren et.al., (Eds.). *Human aging: A biological and behavioral study.* Public Health Services Publication, No. 986, Washington, DC.

Reiter, M.A. (1981). Effects of a physical exercise program on selected mood states in a group of women over age 65. (Doctoral dissertation, Columbia University Teachers College.) *Dissertation Abstracts International, 42,* 1974 A.

Rosenberg, M. (1977). *Sixty-plus and fit again.* New York: M. Evans.

FOOTNOTES

Requests for reprints may be sent to Rayma K. Beal, Ed.D., Department of Health, Physical Education and Recreation, University of Kentucky, Lexington, Kentucky 40506.

12

Folk Dance And The Older Adult

Graham Hempel

The benefits of physical activity for the older adult are clear: maintaining an appropriate level of physical activity in later life leads to better health, greater awareness, and an increased sense of worth. Dance is a beneficial physical activity not only at all age levels but especially for the older adult. Dance promotes cardio-vascular health, reduces stress and anxiety, and encourages social interaction. As social isolation becomes a problem in later years it is even more important to provide opportunities for group interaction. According to Levinton and Santoro (1980), "Dance promotes group interaction and sociability. It recognizes each senior citizen as a valuable person, provides a creative outlet, and improves functional capacities" (p. 117).

Folk dancing provides both the physical activity and the social outlet needed by those who because of their age, find it difficult to maintain either. Folk dance provides an atmosphere of social interaction that is congenial, supportive, and rewarding. Folk dancing has been found to be an appropriate physical activity because each individual can set their own pace by choosing to do only slow dances, or slow and some moderately paced dances, or even a strenuous one now and then. In other words, the individual may sit out those dances they do not want to do and still not feel excluded from the group as there will be other individuals in a similar situation and this is considered to be acceptable behavior.

While there may be very little physical skill required of the beginner, there is also plenty of opportunity to advance to higher levels of skill competency if desired by advancing to more complicated and strenuous dances. Dances that are appropriate for seniors come from all levels and categories of folk dance. Folk dances that have been found to be popular among older adults come form a diverse assortment of cultural backgrounds, range from beginning to advanced in level of complexity, and are easy to moderately difficult in exertion level. Nearly all of the dances that are preferred by seniors are also found to be popular among dancers of differing ages within the recreational folk dance movement. It is this very popularity of these dances that not only can, but does, lead to intergenerational enjoyment of this activity.

The recreational folk dance movement in the United States is a dance movement which welcomes, and is responsive to the needs of, all people of all ages, races, and backgrounds. Recreational folk dancing can be traced back to the early twentieth century, but its increase in popularity as a movement got its biggest boost after World War II with the return of many servicemen from abroad. Some of the people who started folk dancing as a hobby in the late 1940's and early 1950's are still dancing today, forty years later! Have all of the older adults who are currently folk dancing been dancing for forty years or have some of them taken up the activity more recently? Do they dance frequently or rarely? What types of dances do they prefer? In an effort to answer these and other questions about older adults who folk dance, surveys were designed and conducted in 1981 and 1986.

The 1986 Survey

Description of the Population

The population in the 1986 study consisted of fifty men and women over the age of sixty-five who were present at folk dance events. These gatherings took place in, and around the vicinity of, San Diego, California, during weekday afternoons and evenings, and also on weekend afternoons. Five different groups were observed. The number of seniors at each event ranged from four to eighteen with the mean being ten. The events varied from one-and-a-half hour long classes to three hour dance parties, and were held in a variety of facilities such as school auditoriums and a park and recreation department building.

Description of the Activity

The activity that these seniors engaged in consisted of dancing to recordings of folk music from a wide variety of countries. The folk dances that were done were, in most cases, learned from the individual who functioned as dance leader, teacher, and program director. The dances included both couple dances (those that are done with a partner) and line dances (those that are done without a partner). The dances originated primarily in Europe and North America. The types of movements employed were walking, hopping, small leaps, skipping, pivoting, stamping, and occasionally squatting. Those movements were done in both even and uneven rhythms, and a varying tempos. The dances required very little extension of the legs, only small amounts of rotation and flexion of the torso, and moderate to little use of the arms.

The Survey

A single page questionnaire was distributed to all folk dancers at each of the events observed. The questionnaires asked them to choose categories that indicated their age, how many years they've been folk dancing, their gender, their skill level, how often they usually dance, and their reasons for dancing. They were also asked to indicate their five favorite folk dances by name. While all of the dancers at each event were polled, only the data from the seniors was tabulated (in the 1986 survey). It was felt that polling all of the dancers instead of just the seniors would prove to be more successful in collecting data since seniors might feel inhibited about admitting their age if only they were polled.

The number of men and women was 15 and 35 respectively, or 30% men and 70% women. Whencomparing the men to the women, it was evident that most of the men had been dancing for quite a few years(six or more years) while among the women it appeared that a large number were new to folk dancing. More that one half of the women had been dancing for five or fewer years. The reasons for this are unclear; it may have been due to retirement, recent widowhood, or some other factor.

Have people who have been dancing for quite a number of years progresses to more advanced levels of skill? Everyone surveyed was asked to indicate their skill level. As might be expected, people who had danced for less than two years considered themselves to be beginners, those who have danced for two to eleven years rated themselves as intermediates, those who had danced between eleven and twenty years ranked themselves intermediate and advanced, and nearly all of those who have danced for over twenty years considered themselves to be advanced.

How often they folk dance was the next concern. The results indicated that the men danced about as frequently as the women. Nearly two-thirds of all seniors polled danced more that once a week. Although is is not known with accuracy how many more times than once a week, personal observations indicate that most of them danced twice a week, with some dancing as often as three and four times a week.

When asked to give their reasons for folk dancing, each person was allowed to choose more than one response. Both the men and the women indicated that "exercise" was an important reason for dancing, but a much higher number of the women chose it than the men (86% of the women as compared to 60% of the men). The men considered the category "to dance" equally as important as the category "exercise" (with 60% of the men choosing each). However, the women felt that "exercise" was a far more important reason to dance than "to dance" for dance's sake (by 86% to 69%). Women favored "meeting people" as a reason to dance much more than the men did (57% of the women compared to 30% of the men). The women felt that "therapy" (which was not defined) was more important as a reason to folk dance than the men felt it was (23% to 7%).

Does dancing for many years lead to an increase in the frequency of participation? To answer this question two groups were compared: Those who had danced for five or less years and those who had danced for eleven or more years. Among the group dancing for eleven or more years, a greater number of people (33%) danced more that once a week than do those who had danced for five or less years (23%). Three possible reasons for this difference include: the longer a person has danced the more skilled and comfortable they become with the activity and therefore finds it pleasurable enough to do more frequently; the longer a person has danced the more strongly the habit has been established; and the longer a person has danced the more that person relies on the activity for socialization.

Is there a difference between these same two groups as to their reasons for folk dancing? The results suggest a definite trend. "Exercise" is far more important to the group that had been dancing for five years or less than any of the other reasons listed. While among the group that had been dancing for eleven years or more, "exercise", "meeting people", and "to dance" were all very important. In fact, among this later group dancing for its own sake was far more important than among the five years or less group. This suggests that because they had built up more skill and were more comfortable with it, they consider dance to be a pleasurable activity and not merely exercise.

The 1981 Survey

In 1981, 461 folk dancers of all ages throughout southern California were surveyed and seniors (age sixty-five and older) numbered fifty-nine (13%) of the total. The following tables were derived from that data. Table I lists the twenty-five dances found to be the most popular with the older adults in that 1981 survey. The number of people who listed the dance as one of their favorite five dances is indicated under N. The dances have been ranked by frequency, but where there are several dances with the same N they have been arranged alphabetically. Also listed alongside each dance is its nationality, type, and degree of difficulty by complexity and by exertion level.

TABLE I

THE 25 MOST POPULAR FOLK DANCES AMONG THE 65 YEARS AND OLDER AGE GROUP (N=59)

N	DANCE	NATIONALITY	TYPE	DEGREE OF DIFFICULTY COMPLEXITY	EXERTION
13	Hambo	Sweden	cpl	adv	mod-stren
12	Tango	Argentina	cpl	bg-in	easy
8	Haisapiko	Greece	line	int	easy
6	Ada's Kujawiak #3	Poland	cpl	int	mod
5	Polharrow Burn	Scotland	cpl	adv	mod
5	Santa Rita	Mexico	cpl	adv	mod
4	Csardas Z	Hungary	cpl	adv	mod
4	Folsom Prison Blues	USA	cpl	int	easy
4	Miserlou	Greek-Amer.	line	beg	easy
4	Somewhere My Love	USA	cpl	int	easy
4	St. Bernard's Waltz	England	cpl	beg	easy
4	Zillertaler Laendl.	Germany	cpl	int	easy
3	Ali Pasa	Turkey	line	beg	easy
3	Belasichko Oro	Yugoslavia	line	int	mod
3	Couple Haisapiko	Greece	cpl	beg	easy
3	Hofbrauhaus Laendl.	Germany	cpl	int	mod
3	Hopak	Ukraine	cppl	adv	stren
3	Korobushka	Russ.-Amer.	cpl	beg	mod
3	La Bastringue	French-Can.	cpl	beg	easy
3	Russian Sher	Jewish	cpl	int	mod
3	Salty Dog Rag	USA	cpl	beg	mod-stren
3	Sauerlander Quad.	Germany	cpl	int	easy
3	Syrto	Greece	line	int	mod
3	Trip to Bavaria	Scotland	cpl	int	mod
3	Tzadik Katamar	Israel	line	beg	easy

cpl -- couple dance
adv -- advanced
mod-stren -- moderately strenuous
beg -- beginner
int -- intermediate

Table I contains a wide variety of folk dances. Although most of the dances on this list are from Europe and North America, they represent a generous assortment of nationalities. There are a large predominance of couple dances, a good balance in the range of difficulty by complexity, and a high predominance of dances with an easy and moderate exertion level.

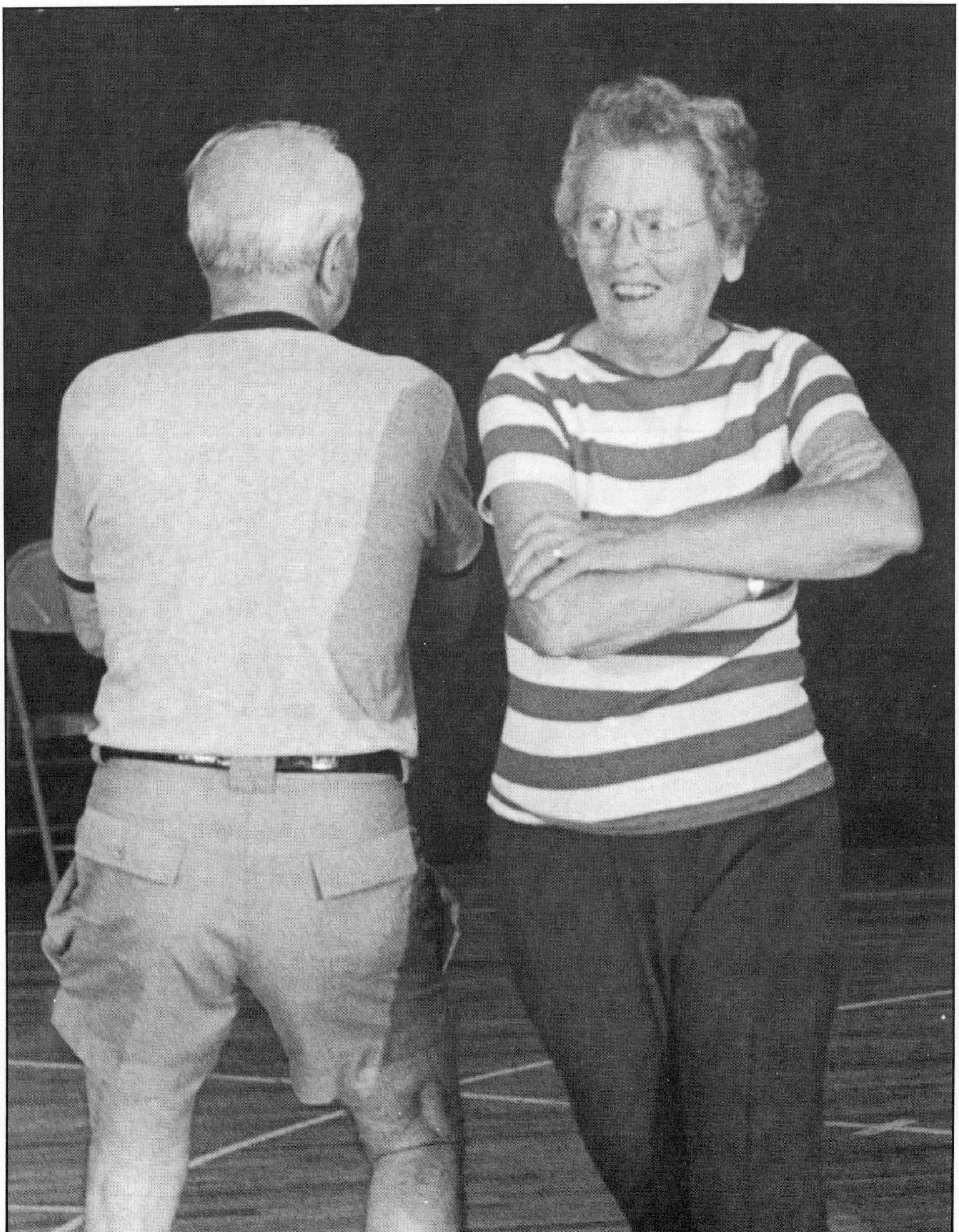

PHOTO COURTESY OF MARIANNE MCADAM

Folk dance provides an atmosphere of social interaction that is congenial, supportive, and rewarding.

Table I also indicates the type of folk dances preferred by the older adults. It is quite evident that seniors prefer couple dances over line dances. Nineteen of the twenty-five most popular dances are couple dances while only six are line dances. The reason for this may be that line dances have always been less popular with this particular generation of folk dancers. When some of them started dancing forty years ago, line dances hadn't arrived on the scene yet. Line dances started appearing (a a barely tolerated appendage to folk dance festivals) in the early 1950's. Line dances were found to be more popular among the younger age groups.

Table 2 compares seniors who had been dancing for over twenty years with those who had been dancing less than twenty years.

TABLE 2

SIXTY FIVE YEARS AND OLDER AGE GROUP

DANCING LESS THAN 20 YEARS (N=29)	N	DANCING MORE THAN 20 YEARS (N=30)	N
Tango	7	Hambo	9
Polharrow Burn	5	Tango	5
Haisapiko	4	Haisapiko	4
Hambo	4	Ada's Kujawiak #3	3
Miserlou	4	Hofbrauhaus Laendler	3
Ada's Kujawiak #3	3	St. Bernard's Waltz	3
Belasichko Oro	3	Sauerlander Quadrille	3
La Bastringue	3	Zillertaler Laendler	3
Russian Sher	3	Ali Pasa	2
Santa Rita	3	Bal in der Stradt	2
Somewhere My Love	3	Corrido	2
Tzadik Katamar	3	Couple Haisapika	2
Black Forest Mazurka	2	Csardas Z	2
Csardas Z	2	Divchibarsko	2
Folsom Prison Blues	2	Elizabeth Quadrille	2
Salty Dog Rag	2	Folsom Prison Blues	2
Syrto	2	Hopak	2
		Korobushka	2
		La Cumparsita	2
		Paso Doble	2
		Polka Mazurka	2
		Santa Rita	2
		Trip to Bavaria	2
		White Heather Jig	2

The group that had been dancing for over twenty years knew a greater number of dances and particularly intermediate level dances of a moderate exertion level. They also had a somewhat different repertoire than the less-than-twenty-years group. For example, they ranked the advanced and moderately strenuous dance Hambo higher then the other group, and they listed the advanced and very strenuous dance Hopak while the group that has been dancing for less than twenty years didn't list it at all.

Perhaps the most significant difference between the two groups is in their preference, or lack of preference, for line dances. The preference for couple dances is greatest with the group that had been dancing for more than twenty years (87% for couple to 13% for line dances). While the other group prefers couple dances to line dances, the difference isn't as great (71% couple to 29% line).

Implications and Recommendations

When setting up a program of instruction or dancing for older adults it is important to make an assessment of the group's variables. Variables such as the structure of the group, skill levels, range of experiences, fitness levels, and range of purposes must be taken into account before designing the program. Structurally, the group might be mixed evenly between men and women, contain more women that men (the usual case), or be an all women's group. Skill levels could range from beginner in a group that was taking up folk dancing for the first time to advanced in a group with a lot of previous experience; however, a typical group would probably contain many levels of skills. A group's range of experiences may vary, according to their socio-economic and educational background, from no dance experience and very little exposure to foreign cultures to a lot of familiarity with dance and a very strong appreciation for other people's cultures. Although fitness levels usually don't vary too widely in most groups, the instructor may occasionally be faced with having to accommodate a disparity of levels. The range of purposes for engaging in the activity often varies greatly, with some seniors desiring exercise, some wanting to meet people, and others having a variety of reasons for wanting to folk dance.

After having determined the group's structure, background, and needs the teacher may select dances for a plan of instruction. The dances should match the group's needs as closely as possible. A fairly even ratio between men and women might necessitate the use of more couple dances than line dances (especially if they were all married couples who wanted to dance with their spouses), while a group containing many women and few men would suggest a liberal use of trio dances (utilizing two women and one man). An all women's group might indicate the use of line dances perhaps even to the exclusion of couple dances. The use of line dances is very important in any instructional program in folk dance, particularly at the beginner level. Line dances don't involve working with a partner and therefore make it easier for the students to concentrate on their own steps and styling. Couple dances are usually more complex as an activity because in addition to the steps and styling the dancer must coordinate their movements with those of their partner and learn to utilize leading and following techniques. It is important to include line dances when the group contains many singles, and especially when it contains no men.

The primary consideration in dance selection is the ability level of the students. Dance students must be made to feel that they're succeeding and making progress. This can be facilitated by the establishment of a logical and meaningful teaching progression.

A teaching progression for an all beginners class should start with only beginning level dances and then leisurely advance to slightly more difficult dances. Simple line dances should be chosen at first and then some mixers and simple couple dances can be gradually added. Mixers, couple dances in which the dancer progresses from one partner to another, are wonderful icebreakers that provide the opportunity for everyone to relax and get to meet everyone else. More difficult line dances and complex couple dances can be added into the teaching progression as the students gain more skill and confidence.

Only dances with even musical rhythms should be employed, as dances with uneven rhythms are too overwhelming for the beginner. Dances that contain simple, alternating weight changes (such as walking) are much easier to use initially than dances with hops, jumps, and leaps. The least strenuous dances should be chosen first (especially if there is a predominance of unfit people in the group and more strenuous ones added gradually. In order to maintain student interest, a variety of dances should be included that make use of an assortment of tempos, changing dynamics in movements, steps, and styling. Dances may be modified to facilitate learning if the teacher accepts the responsibility for returning the dance to its original state of authenticity at some time shortly after the students develop the appropriate skill. As an example, if a dance contains both complex foot and arm movements that arm movements can be neutralized, while the students concentrate on the foot movements, and then added in later. All of the previous recommendations have been combined with the data from Table I (The 25 Most Popular Folk Dances) to produce a suggested teaching progression for a class of older adults at the beginning level. That progression is shown here in Table 3.

TABLE 3

SAMPLE TEACHING PROGRESSION FOR BEGINNING LEVEL OLDER ADULTS

1	Ail Pasa
2	Miserlou
3	Tango
4	Couple Haisapiko
5	Tzadik Katamar
6	St. Bernard's Waltz
7	LaBastringu
8	Korobushka
9	Haisapiko
10	Salty Dog Rag

A teaching progression for a class of seniors of mixed ability levels necessitates all of the prior considerations plus the incorporation of a wider assortment of folk dances to include a mixture of levels proportionate to the skill levels of the seniors involved, a better balance between line, mixer, and couple dances, the admission of a few dances with uneven musical rhythms, the inclusion of more difficult and complex dances, and the addition of a few strenuous ones. The foregoing principles also apply to programming a recreational folk dance event with, additionally, the inclusion of the widest possible assortment of dances and making use of contrasts such as alternating line dances with couple dances, slow dances with fast ones, and easy dances with strenuous ones.

Summary

Folk dancing is beneficial to the older adult both physically and socially. Folk dance teachers can structure classes to enhance these benefits by assessing, and meeting, the varying needs of the older adult. Folk dancing is one of the many physical activities that the older adult may choose to assist themselves in maintaining health, and one in which they may choose their own level of involvement. Recent surveys have revealed that a number of people who folk dance are over the age of sixty-five; that many of these older adults have been folk dancing for a long time and go folk dancing more than once a week; that still other seniors have taken up folk dancing just recently; that they dance for a variety of reasons but primarily for exercise, to enjoy dancing, and to meet people; and that the more years a person has danced the more frequently they will go dancing. The survey results have produced a listing of the twenty-five folk dances most favored by the older adult. Recommendations for designing teaching progression and a recreational program for seniors include assessing group variables and selection of dances.

REFERENCES

Harris, J.A., Pittman, A.M., & Waller, M.S. (1978). Dance a while: Handbook of folk, square, and social dance. (5th ed.). Minneapolis, MN: Burgess.

Hayes, E.R. (1964). An introduction to the teaching of dance. New York: Ronald Press.

Hempel, G. (1982, October). The top 51: A survey of dance favorites. Folk Dance Scene, 10, pp. 6-7.

Kraus, R. (1962). Folk dancing: A guide for schools, colleges, and recreational groups. New York: MacMillan.

Leviton, D.,& Santoro, L.C. (Eds.). (1980). Health, Physical Education, Recreation and Dance for the older adult: A modular approach. Reston, VA : AAHPERD.

Smith, E.L. & Serfass, R.C. (Eds.). (1981). Exercise and aging: The scientific basis. Hillside, NJ: Enslow.

Snider, M.E. (1980). Folk dance: Handbook. Vancouver, B.C.: Hancock House.

AUTHOR NOTES

Further details of the results can be obtained by writing the author at the Department of Physical Education, San Diego State University, San Diego, CA 92182-0171.

13

Dance Movement: Effects on Elderly Self-Concept

Sherrill Berryman-Miller

Contrary to popular belief, older adults have a highly developed sense of kinesthetic connection. Dance activities are unique in exploiting that awareness. Dance presents a vocabulary of simple movements in isolation. For example, an older adult can analyze a stiff elbow by observing the action of his or her glenohumeral joint. Isolated movements can be transformed into rhythmic sequences which lead not opnly to improved movement, but to a better sense of the body in space.

Through a study conducted at Howard University, in Washington, DC, I sought to explore the effects of self-concept in older adults. The short-term goal was a rediscovery of pleasure in movement. This enjoyment should grow into physical fitness in two stages. First, older adults learn to move with confidence. Second, they participate in activities with others. Through these activities, aspects of self-awareness begin to evolve as they did during the first three years of life: a sense of bodily self, a sense of continuing self-identity, and a sense of self-esteem and pride.

The long-term goal was to motivate the aging person to "move within the principles of efficient human motion." This involves not only physical but psychological adjustment. Toward this end people must begin to view their own bodies objectively. Then they will begin to understand that attention to their own needs is not selfish but prudent, and that the time and effort spent in exercise improves the body immediately and over time. An underlying message for the older adult is that the responsibilities of self-care are a part of retirement. A retired person who must abandon the work ethic may replace it with a conscientious concern for health and independence.

Research design and methods

The study measured the effect of regular classes in dance/movement on the self-concept of the retired, healthy older adult. A comparative descriptive methodology was used. A pretest questionnaire sought information about personal characteristics, exercises, and social participation patterns. The Tennessee Self-Concept Scale Questionnaire was used as a posttest. The scale was normed on a sample of 626 persons of varying age, sex, race, and socioeconomic status. Retest reliability and validity was in the high .80's.

A dance educator served as principal investigator. She selected university students from the areas of Dance and Physical Medicine and Rehabilitation at Howard University. They worked with an experimental group of older adults from The Senior Citizens Counseling and Delivery Center, in Washington, D.C. A control group was identified at the Columbia Senior Center, Also in Washington, D.C. The continued participation of experimental Group A in dance/movement classes was compared to the noninvolvement of control Group B to measure the effect of dance/movement classes on the self-concept of the retired, healthy older adult. The participants in the experimental groups engaged in eight months of biweekly classes in dance/movement. Sessions ran for an hour and a half. Each session was carefully planned to include a general warmup, a sequence of dance movements done while sitting, standing, and locomoting, a special focus of the particular day, and cooling-down activities. Before the project began, the university students participated in orientation and training sessions to acquaint themselves with class format and activities.

In orientation, the student group discussed proper screening of all new movement students as well as particular precautions for working with older adults. Factors addressed included:

1. Risk factor assessment--Information received from a doctor; results from electrocardiograms; ongoing medical assessments

2. Past athletic participation

3. Individual weight

4. Existence of hypertension

5. Smoking history

The university students were required to have training in cardiopulmonary resuscitation techniques (CPR) for certification by the American Red Cross as well as sessions in how to monitor heart rates and identify signs of exertional intolerance (dizziness, angina, nausea, respiratory difficulty, and unusuall fatigue or pain.

Subjects

Adult men and women, between the ages of 55 and 85, were recruited from senior centers in southeast and northwest Washington, D.C. Participants were selected with caution; written *approval* from a physician was solicited. Physicians were asked to list both precautions and recommended activities for each patient.

The Dance/Movement Program was designed to minimize risks for participants. The design incorporated guidelines suggested by the 1987 American Alliance Committee on Aging.

A typical class includes warm-up movements in a chair. The participants prepared for the movements by moving forward to the front edge of the seat. They began with a two-minute deep breathing routine. Using a stopwatch to monitor the procedure, the participants were instructed to feel the tiny pulsating movements at the wrist or throat and to count their own "resting pulse." They were asked to stand up and sit down repeatedly for one nimute. Each combination took four seconds: two to stand, two to sit. The group leader says: "Breathe in to stand, breathe out to sit." The combined breathing and stand-and-sit movements were performed fifteen times in the minute. This alternative to the customary shallow breathing of most older adults helps relax the bodies for movement.

The ensuing 10 minutes were devoted to warm-up movements which start with the facial and neck muscles and advance to arms, hands, torso, back, abdominal, anterior/posterior thigh, leg and foot muscles. These warm-ups increase the degree of mobility at each of the joints.

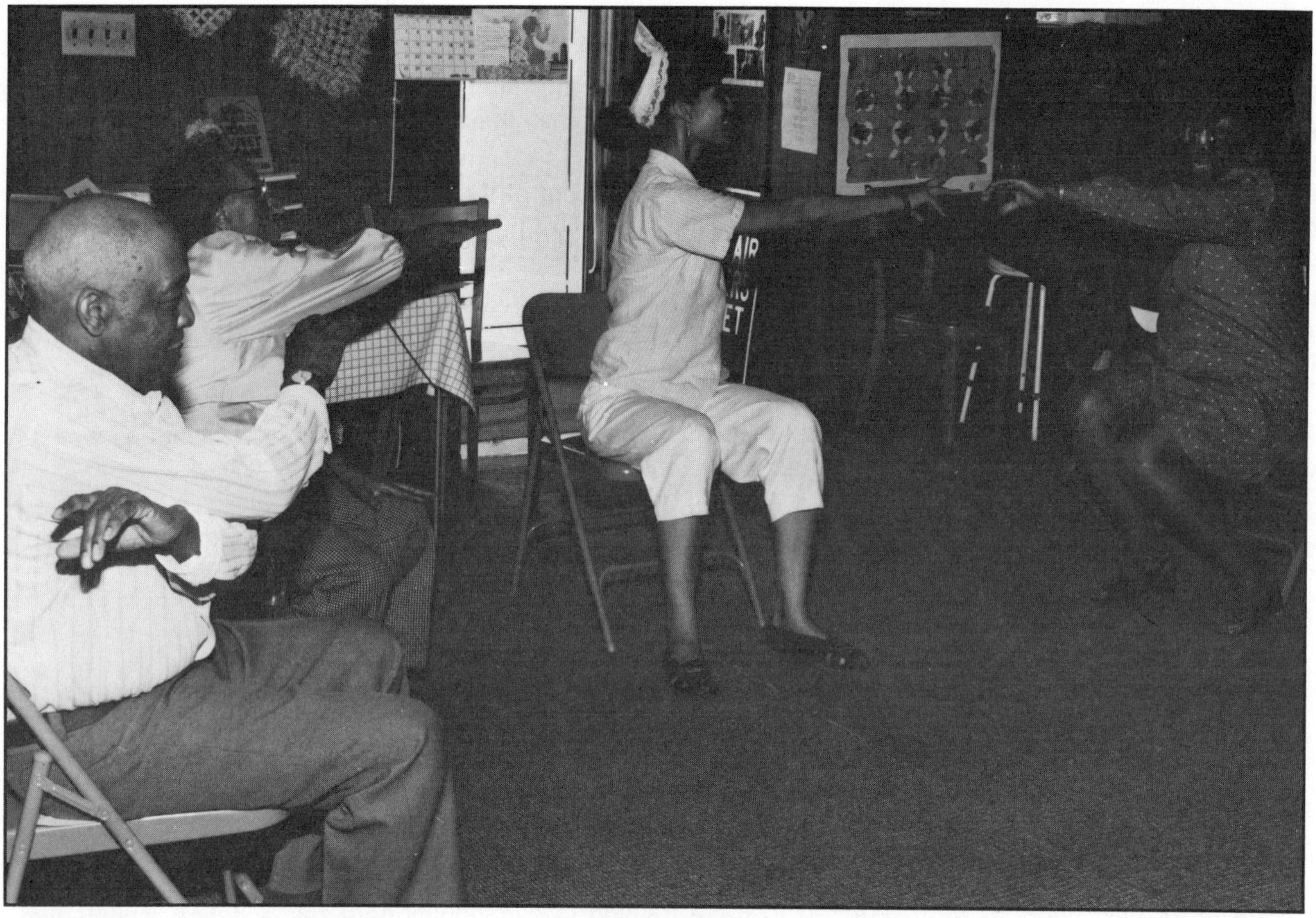
PHOTO COURTESY OF ANDRE RICHARDSON

This project led to increased creativity, cooperation, and interaction in the student-adult relationship.

Table 1. Mean Scores and 2-Tail Probability Comparing Experimental Group to the Control Group on Responses to 29 Tennessee Concepts

Scale Items

		Experimental	Control	Probability
1.	Healthy body	4.31	2.16	0.000
2.	An attractive person	4.04	2.58	0.000
3.	A decent sort of person	4.43	3.77	0.025
4.	A cheerful person	4.30	3.65	0.012
5.	A calm and easygoing person	4.43	3.81	0.014
6.	Have a family that would always help me	4.39	3.23	0.000
7.	Member of a happy family	4.43	3.04	0.000
8.	A friendly person	4.39	3.42	0.001
9.	A religious person	4.59	4.00	0.044
10.	A lot of self-control	4.23	3.38	0.007
11.	I am an important person to my family and friends	4.13	3.42	0.008
12.	Neither too fat or too thin	3.96	1.92	0.000
13.	I like my looks just the way they are	3.83	2.54	0.001
14.	Satisfied with my relationship with God	4.70	4.23	0.041
15.	Satisfied to be just what I am	4.26	3.58	0.020
16.	Satisfied with my family relationship	4.52	4.08	0.030
17.	I am as sociable as I want to be	4.17	3.38	0.005
18.	Try to please others, but I don't overdo it	4.00	2.92	0.003
19.	I am as religious as I want to be	4.35	3.54	0.020
20.	At times I feel like swearing	4.00	2.77	0.001
21.	I take good care of myself physically	4.04	2.69	0.001
22.	I try to be careful about my appearance	4.13	3.23	0.007
23.	I try to understand the other fellow's point of view	4.09	3.38	0.010
24.	I feel good most of the time	3.96	2.92	0.003
25.	I do what is right most of the time	4.26	3.62	0.005
26.	I do my share of work at home	4.35	3.42	0.001
27.	I see good points in all people	4.04	3.00	0.000
28.	I am true to my religion every day	4.35	3.50	0.005
29.	I try to change when I am doing wrong	4.30	3.54	0.006

After warm-ups, 15 to 20 minutes of rhythmic tempo movement with vocalization were performed to music. Emphasis was on a relaxed, flowing and swinging type of movement repeated on either side of the body with complete body freedom.

One third of the class time was reserved for relaxing and vitalizing techniques. These techniques enhanced the awareness of muscle and joint interaction. The relaxing techniques were adapted from motor responses surrendering to gravity. The vitalizing techniques were achieved mostly through rhythmic movements which oppose gravity. Other techniques in this category included extremely mild isometric contractions.

In class, group leaders used the vocabulary of dance: fall, rebound, swing, and suspension. These dance terms signify movement responses to gravity. Such maneuvers require the conscious involvement of participants. For example, the term "succession" refers to a pattern of coordinated movements that progress along adjacent muscles and joints. The moving parts must first be controlled individually before they can be moved sequentially. The student group leaders were instructed to use this and other terms since it would awaken self-consciousness in the participants.

During their training, the student group leaders were encouraged to use creativity and to recognize creativity in participants. In addition, improvisation was explored. Through improvisation, for example, a group leader could discover how many ways, and in what positions, each participant could straighten and bend knees. Group leaders, in offering individual attention, discovered that no two participants moved in the same way. Group leaders presented simple movements to the class and asked participants to suggest variations. The group leaders would add a beginning and an end to the improvised movement to create a brief composition which could be performed by the class.

The student group leaders conducted classes as a team. While one was conducting class, the other would use a checklist to monitor the class format, individual involvement of the participants, as well as the group responses.

Results

At the of eight months the researcher calculated mean scores and performed t-tests to determine significant self-concept differences between the experimental and control group of older adults. At the .05 level of significance, findings (summarized in Table 1) were observed for the experimental group. The items recorded in Table 2 indicate significant differences ($p < .05$) for the control group's low level of self-concept.

The mean scores reflecting the experimental group's sense of personal worth, feelings of adequacy as individuals, personality apart from the body and relationships to others are evidence that in the adult aging process, a sense of control, respect and valued identity must be maintained. These attitudes, experts say, seem to be primary in regulating one's quality of life and perhaps one's longevity as well.

In Table 2, the rather high rates reported by the control group reflect the significance of personality characteristics in the relationship between activity and morale. Another factor is the extent to which social networks encourage or discourage participation.

It is becoming increasingly clear that aging in humans is not simply a biological process, but rather a "biopsychosocial" process in which changes in social environment and psychological dispositions, as well as genetic factors, are involved. Evidence is accumulating that there is no single cause for aging. Thus from a variety of psychological and social perspectives, research must seriously investigate the influence of diverse activities on the aging process.

Conclusions

The most evident and significant conclusion to be drawing from this research is that a dance/movement class will influence the positive image of self-concept for the older adult. Accoring to the results of the t-test, the experimental group possessed stronger self-concept in the areas of physical self and personal self.

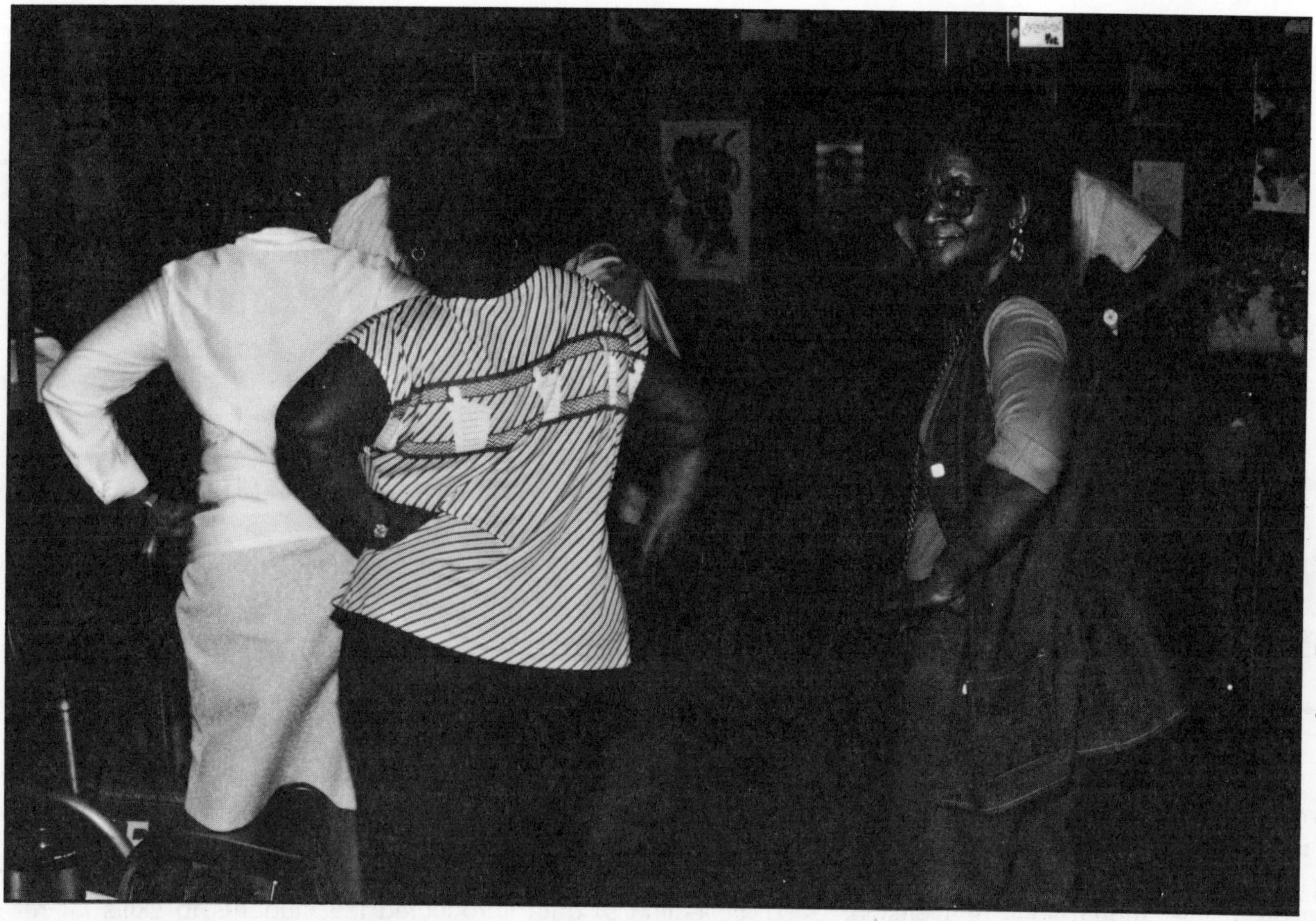

PHOTO COURTESY OF ANDRE RICHARDSON

Dance/movement programs improve self-esteem and rekindle *joie de vivre*.

TABLE 2. Mean Scores and 2-Tail Probability Reflecting Control Group and Experimental Group Responses to 9 Tennessee Concept Scale

		Mean Score		2-Tail Probability
		Control	Experiemental	
1.	I am a nobody	2.04	1.04	0.000
2.	My friends have no confidence in me	2.19	1.39	0.005
3.	I am full of aches and pains	3.88	2.09	0.000
4.	I am a sick person	3.54	2.04	0.000
5.	I am not loved by my family	2.08	1.26	0.005
6.	I am hard to be friendly with	2.46	1.57	0.003
7.	I despise myself	2.00	4.52	0.018
8.	I don't feel as well as I should	3.31	2.52	0.038
9.	I would like to change some part of my body	3.23	2.35	0.045

Positive benefits to both students and participants emerged from the study. Intergenerational probing between students and older adults about *what* they were observing and *how* to correct movement problems led to a heightened awareness of individual joint and muscle usage and body habits. Both groups began to view their bodies in ways that had been unexplored. This project led to increased creativity, cooperation and interaction in the student-adult relationship. Also, collecting of data introducted the students to skills for research.

While some service programs are funded, relatively little research has been conducted in these areas, either because of low priority or because of limited resources. Yet the importance of these services increases with the growth of the population segment in retirement. As the over-65 population continues to increase, the implementation of dance/movement programs for improving self-esteem and rekindling *joie de vivre* must be tailored to service the needs of this group.

REFERENCES

American Alliance Committee on Aging. (1981, October 2-4). Guidelines for Exercise Programs for Older Persons (Age 50 and older) Addendum B-1. *Official Minutes: Board of Governors,* AAHPERD.

IV. Curricular Program Models

14

Age Doesn't Matter

Weaving Dance And Aging Into A Fifth Grade Curriculum

Josie Metal-Corbin, David E. Corbin, And Gwyn Barker

Aging is a part of living, as natural as life itself, yet many people tend to view aging negatively. Stereotypical attitudes about aging are prevalent in the adult population and have also been identified in children. How children view their own aging appears to have serious implications for society. Children who hold negative attitudes toward aging may disassociate themselves from older people. Surveys in recent years have indicated that a majority of children have negative attitudes toward older adults and toward the idea of getting older themselves (Jantz, Seefeldt, Galper, & Serock, 1977; Olivas, Driver & Driver, 1981). Children generally described older persons as lonely, bored, grouchy, uninterested in life, and inactive -- a stereotypical image of physical degeneration. Only 22% of the 180 children surveyed by Jantz et al. (1977) could name an older person outside of their family. These surveys indicate that children have very limited contact with older adults. Children's negative attitudes may be a function of this lack of personal contact with older people.

Survey data concerning attitudes toward older adults confirm the general principle that attitudes are formed early in life and they tend to endure (Klausmeier & Ripple, 1971). By the age of eight, most children have well-defined negative attitudes toward older persons and toward the aging process (Hickey, Hickey, & Kalish, 1968). By adolescence, most of the negative characteristics stereotypically associated with old age appear firmly established (Kastenbaum & Durkee, 1964).

In view of the fact that about 12% of Americans are over age 65 and 13% of the population will be over 65 by the year 2000, it seems critical that our society examine how we are preparing children to adjust to their own aging and their parents' aging. "The best time to learn about growing old with decency and grace is in youth," according to a study conducted by Gerbner, Gross, Morgan and Signorielli (1981) at the Annenburg School of Communications at the University of Pennsylvania.

Educators, researchers, sociologists, gerontologists, and artists must explore what Betty Friedan calls the "mystique of age" if American society is to produce an image of aging that is not completely negative. How can we confront agism and develop new ways of looking at and reacting to growing older? How can we break through the stereotypes and misunderstandings that abound in the public eye? One of the best ways to change

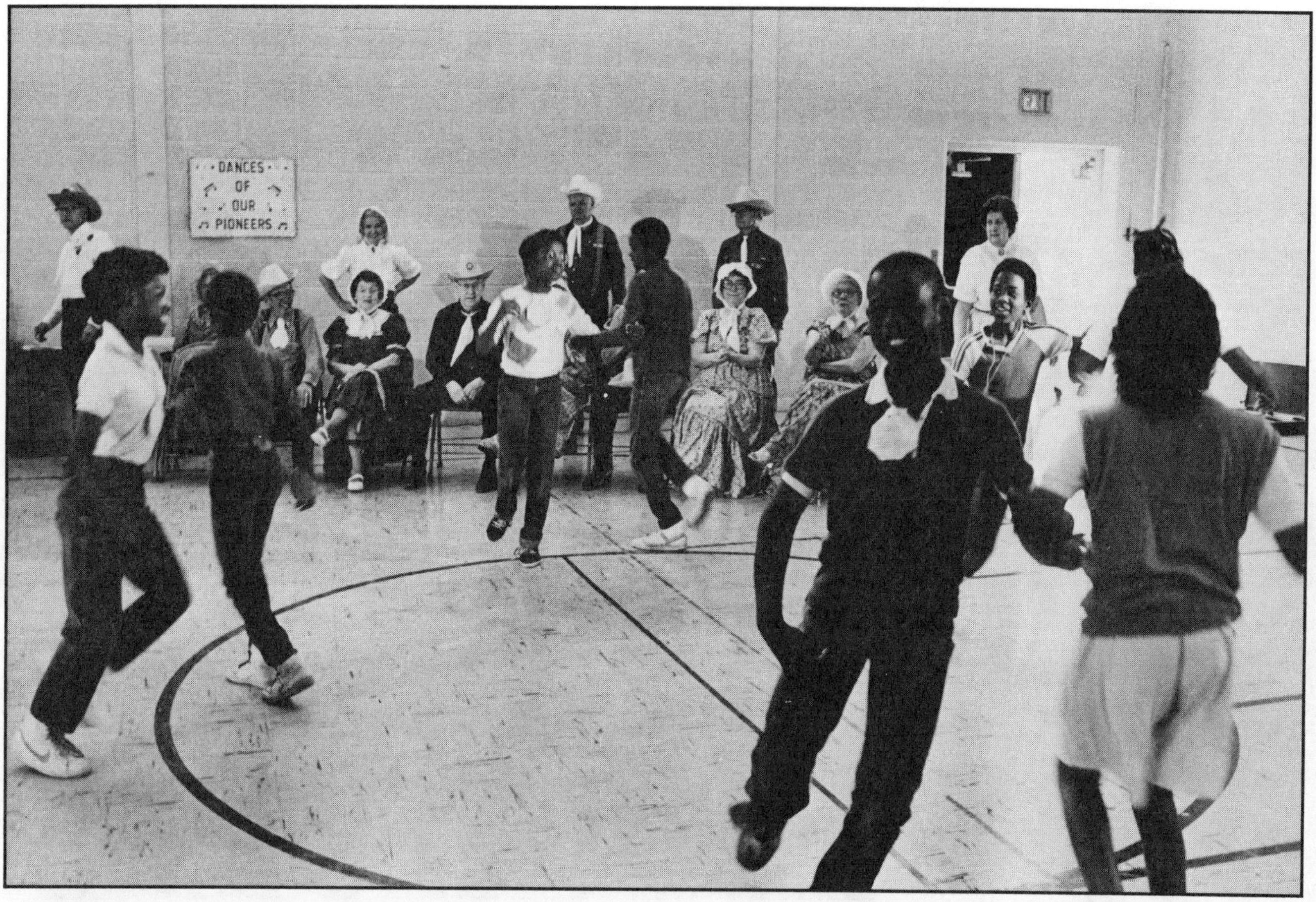

PHOTO COURTESY OF DAVID E. CORBIN

The ADM program at Mt. View showed that the schools can have a role in helping to break down age ghettos and putting people of all ages in touch with each other.

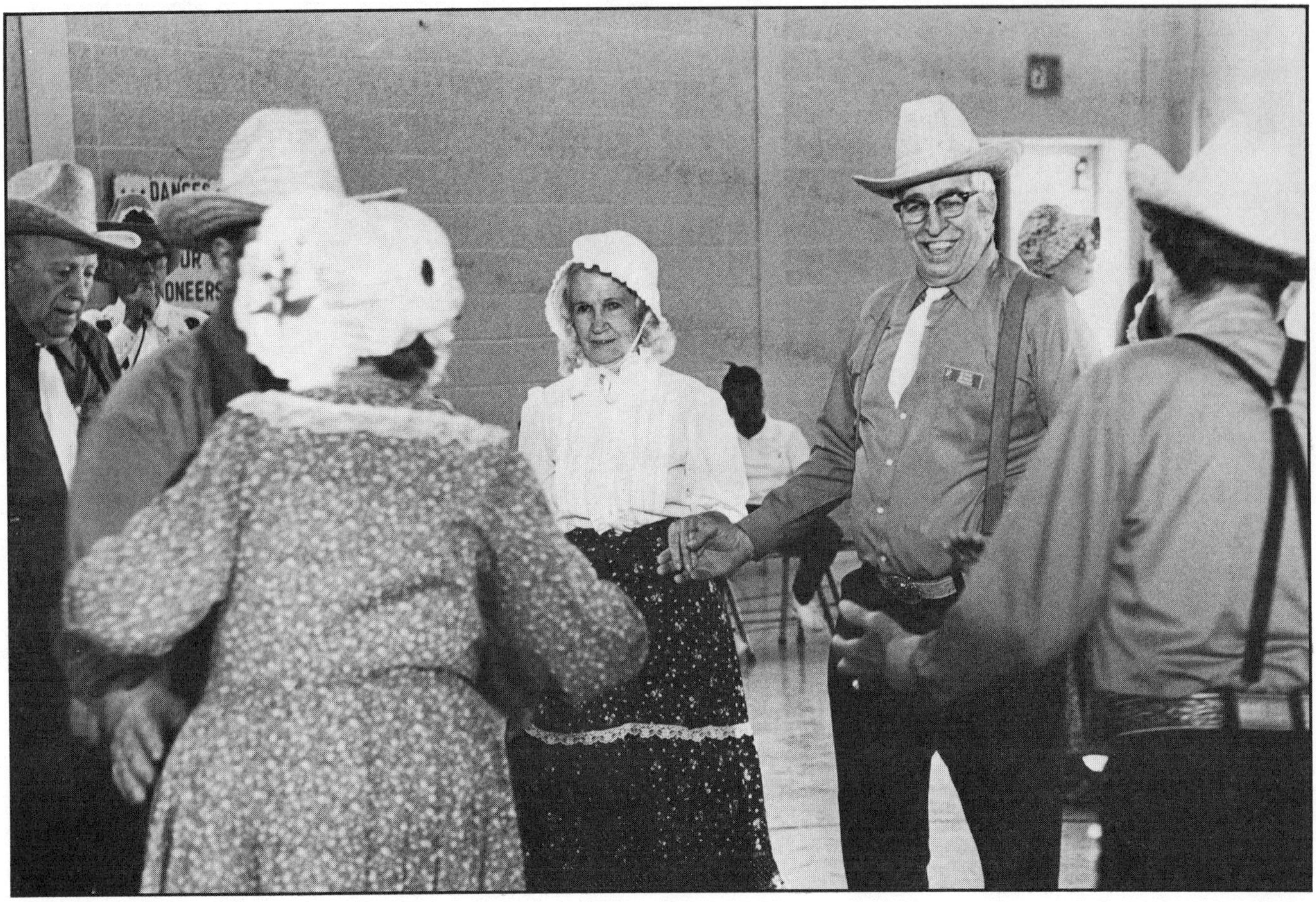

PHOTO COURTESY OF DAVID E. CORBIN

The students and the "Sodbusters" quickly learned that one way to bring generations together was through dance.

stereotypical attitudes is through repeated personal relationships which allow different groups to see each other as unique individuals (Merrill, 1961). This is the rationale behind a current movement to bring education and experiential learning about older people into the elementary public schools, before negative attitudes become fixed. Frymier's extensive survey in 1979 indicated that 73% of elementary schools offered no education at all on aging.

Project Philosophy and Description

We have no reason to believe that our society's tendency to segregate the old from the young can do anything but deprive each generation of important pieces of its past and its future. Buck (1967) said: ". . . the child should be taught from the very first that the whole world is his world, that adult and child share one world, that all generations are needed." Secunda (1984) stated that " . . . each generation is required to give its members an ongoing collective sense of worth they cannot get separately." McGuire (1987) said that:

> "Aging education should be integrated routinely into schools' curricula. It must be intergenerational, developmentally focused, anticipatory education that promotes positive attitudes toward age and aging. It involves cognitive knowledge, but emphasizes the affective domain of learning."

In May of 1985, a seven day project called "Age Doesn't Matter" (ADM) integrated aging into a fifth-grade curriculum with a special emphasis on dance at an elementary school in Omaha, Nebraska. An associate professor in dance was the Artist-in-the-Schools and the participating teacher was a veteran of 25 years of elementary school teaching.

The ADM project focused on activities that incorporated concepts of aging into lessons emphasizing dance. The interdisciplinary approach to the project also used art, music, poetry, health education, language arts, and social studies lessons to bring children and older members of the community together to learn about various aspects of aging. Older adults (ranging in age from 50 - 100 years) visited the classroom to take part in the activities and the fifth grade students visited a local retirement hotel and a nursing home. A television crew from KYNE-TV at the University of Nebraska at Omaha was on location throughout the residency to film a documentary of the project (Bottum, Metal-Corbin, Barker & Corbin, 1985).

The ADM residency was a collaborative effort of the Nebraska Arts Council, the School of Health, Physical Education, and Recreation and the College of Education at the University of Nebraska at Omaha, and the Mt. View Parent Teacher Organization.

Focus on Dance

The arts are one avenue for gaining enlightenment on social issues, and the arts can help with the development of a new sensitivity towards aging. Dance was selected as a focal point for integrating aging concepts into the fifth grade curriculum for several reasons: 1) movement is basic to all human beings -- indeed, the underlying philosophy of this project is that dance is for everyone; 2) dance is a lifelong activity that can bring people of all ages together -- it incorporates movement with fun; 3) dance affords people the opportunity to make contact with one another; and 4) creative dance helps people to express themselves in ways other than through speaking and it helps people to break down their inhibitions. (Corbin & Metal-Corbin, 1983). Dance helps to fuse the contrived divisions between mind and body. Capra (1982) suggests that we need "to 'think' with our bodies" and "use them as agents of knowing."

The art of dance with its creative and expressive powers can provide an environment through which people of all ages can communicate past memories and present feelings. According to Missinne & Lorenzen (1982), older people bring the gift of accumulated years of experience and knowledge of the world and themselves to art. "Potentially, they have the most to say about what it means to be human." According to Leonard (1986), "Music and dance, the blending of rhythmic sound with movement, lubricate all learning, and it is tragic that these subjects are considered anything less than basic in our schools."

During the ADM seven day residency, the fifth grade students received at least a one hour lesson in creative dance each day. The lessons included experiences with locomotor movements, shapes, levels, dynamics, time, and space. On five of the seven days, older adults from the community danced with the students. These intergenerational dance activities included social dance, square dance, folk dance, modern dance, and improvisational activities with parachutes, ribbons, scarves, and other props.

One major aspect of ADM was to provide an opportunity for the children to be exposed to a wide diversity of older adults. The children conducted interviews with older adults and found out that dance was, and still is, a part of their lives. Older adult volunteers gave interviews and were recruited from various sources within the community. Contacts were made with organizations ranging from the Eastern Nebraska Office on Aging to the Great Plains Black History Museum to the Grande Olde Players (a theatrical troupe). Classroom speakers included people from the Retired Senior Volunteer Program (RSVP), marathon runners, race walkers, artists, and dancers. When the Sodbusters, a square dance group from Council Bluffs, Iowa came to Mt. View, the students and the Sodbusters quickly learned that one way to bring generations together was to dance together. The differences in ages did not seem to be a barrier to having a good time. When the Sodbusters were through performing and teaching dances, they requested that the Mt. View students demonstrate the dances that they most enjoy. They were treated to a spontaneous exhibition of breakdancing.

Another highlight of the project was a bus trip to Paxton Manor, a retirement hotel in downtown Omaha. In the words of classroom teacher Gwyn Barker: "They had 'neat' things at the Paxton: an old fashioned roomy ladies' room; an antique barber pole; a ceramics workshop; a ballroom; a billiards room; and creaky old elevators. We felt almost adopted."

While at Paxton Manor, the children were entertained by the Paxton Pacers, its goodtime band. The children joined in a sing-along of songs from bygone years. After the singing, old and young participated in some dances in chairs and some rhythmic parachute play. The morning activities ended with a demonstration of ancient Chinese dance-like exercises called t'ai chi ch'uan, as demonstrated by one of the residents who had been taking lessons locally.

A main emphasis of the project was to expose the children to a cross-section of older adults. After visiting with healthy, active, independent older adults at Paxton Manor, the students visited Redman Nursing Home where they were reminded that some older people need special care and attention.

Another part of the project involved making masks in art class. The masks represented someone they admired or someone they would like to be. Said Mrs. Barker: "Our room became a scrap paper paradise. Noses, ears, mouths, teeth, eyes and lashes appeared like magic. Plastic surgery was done with abandon and creativity. Yarn, cotton, and felt assisted in hair restoration. Our blank masks soon had expressions, personality, and unique identities . . ." They symbolized the project's emphasis on diversity of people of all ages.

The last activity of the residency was a celebration. The dance, art, poetry, and journal entries that had taken place throughout the week were performed, displayed or presented to each other and to the guest of honor Aunt Sally Williams -- who was 100 years old. The end of the celebration was a dance "obstacle course" that incorporated the masks and many of the dance movements and dance vocabulary that the children had learned in the creative dance aspect of the project. Through interacting and dancing with older people, the children at Mt. View learned that older people are "Fountains of Information" -- of history, of life, and of what growing old means to them. It became apparent that youth had much to gain from interacting with older people, but it was equally apparent that youth also had much to teach.

The testimonials of both young and old participants were so positive that a one-year follow-up was conducted on the students of this project. The results of the one-year follow-up revealed that the children involved with the ADM project, as blindly judged by gerontology experts, viewed aging as significantly ($p < .05$) more positive than students in the same school and grade level who did not participate in the project (Corbin, Metal-Corbin & Barg, 1988). In May of 1986, a nine-day residency involving sixth graders at

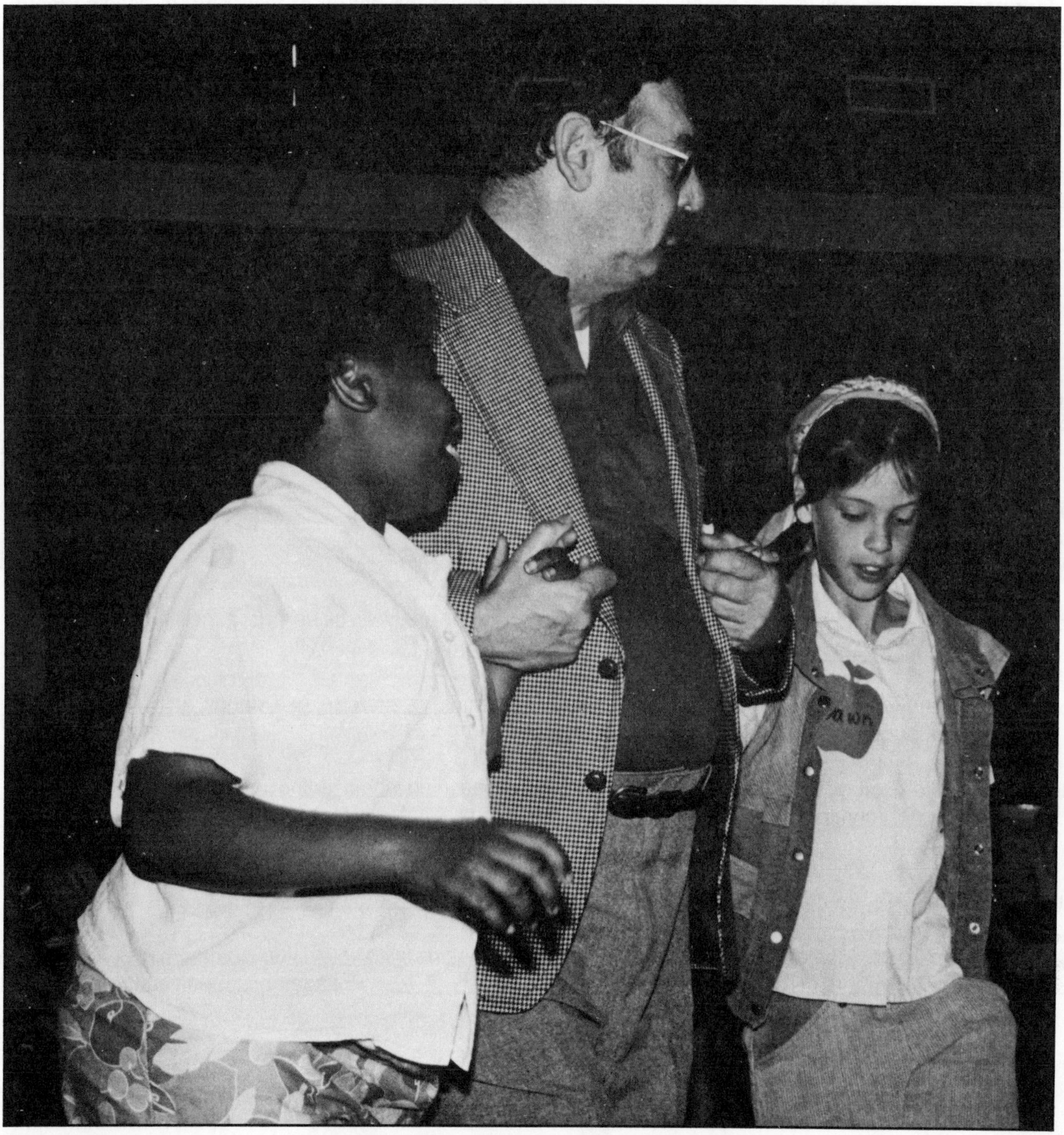

PHOTO COURTESY OF DAVID E. CORBIN

One major aspect of ADM was to provide an opportunity for the children to be exposed to a wide diversity of older adults.

Dundee Elementary School in Omaha was conducted and a multi-perspective content analysis was completed. A short term follow-up of this project suggested that as the program progressed, the children began to perceive the older participants in active rather than passive terms, and that the nature of the program became more interactive (Corbin, Kagan, & Metal-Corbin, 1987).

The intergenerational cooperative ADM program at Mt. View required more than just throwing two or more generations together. In preparation for the actual implementation of this project, the organizers involved parents, community, the principal, librarian, art teacher, and custodian. All of the groundwork began months in advance. The organizers of this project showed that the schools could have a role in helping to break down age ghettos and putting people of all ages in touch with each other -- not solely as caregivers to each other, but as equal partners sharing in all aspects of life with a chance to learn, move, and dance together.

REFERENCES

Bottom, D. (Producer/Director), Metal-Corbin, J., Barker, G. (Project Directors), & Corbin, D. (Narrator/Writer). (1985). Age doesn't matter: Weaving dance and aging into a fifth grade curriculum. [Videotape]. Omaha, NE: University Television, University of Nebraska at Omaha.

Buck, P. (1967). To my daughters, with love. New York: John Day.

Capra, F. (1982). The turning point. New York: Bantam.

Corbin, D.E., Kagan, D.M., & Metal-Corbin, J. (1987). Content analysis of an intergenerational unit on aging in a sixth-grade classroom. Educational Gerontology, 13, 403-410.

Corbin, D.E., Metal-Corbin, J. (1984) Reach for it: A handbook of exercise and dance activities for older adults. Dubuque, IA: Eddie Bowers Publishing Co.

Corbin, D.E., Metal-Corbin, J., & Barg, C. (1988, March). Teaching about aging in the elementary school: A one-year follow-up. Paper presented at the meeting of the American Society on Aging, San Diego, CA

Frymier, R.J. (1979). Aging in the public school. Educational Gerontology, 4, 19-24.

Gerbner, G., Gross, L., Morgan, M. & Signorielli, N. (1981). Aging with television commercials: Images on television commercials and dramatic programming, 1977-79. Philadelphia: University of Pennsylvania, The Annenberg School of Communications.

Hickey, T., Hickey, L., & Kalish, R.A. (1968). Children's perceptions of the elderly. Journal of Genetic Psychology, 112, 227-235.

Jantz, R., Seefeldt, C., Galper, A., & Serock, K. (1977). Children's attitudes toward the elderly. Social Education, 41, 518-523.

Kastenbaum, R. & Durkee, N. (1964). Young people view old age. In R. Kastenbaum (Ed.), New thoughts on old age. (pp. 237-250). New York: Harper & Row.

Leonard, G. (1986). The silent pulse. New York: E.P. Dutton.

McGuire, S.L. (1987). Aging education in schools. Journal of School Health, 57, 174-176.

Merrill, F.E. (1961). Society and culture. Englewood Cliffs, NJ: Prentice-Hall.

Missinne, L. & Lorenzen, L. (1982). The new "wonder drug." Perspectives on Aging, 11, 15.

Olivas, R., Driver, J., & Driver, R. (1981). Children's attitudes toward the elderly and aging. Educational Gerontology, 7, 43-47.

Secunda, V. (1984). By youth possessed. Indianapolis: Bobbs-Merrill.

15

Shared Movement Programs

Children And Older Adults

Erna Caplow Lindner And Leah Harpaz

Rhythmic, creative movement, which is a nonverbal, spontaneous response of the total human being, is an ideal modality for intergenerational communication. Young and old participants in shared movement programs may reap different benefits. Such programs offer the children one to one attention, nonjudgmental acceptance, and patient assistance which may not be available in their school or home. Traditional movement activities from various cultures and even history may be taught to children through the reminiscences of the older group members. The youngsters may also develop more positive views of aging. For the older generation, contacts with children evoke delight and rekindled interest in the present and the future. The shared activities are often eagerly anticipated and the raised energy levels and increased physical participation offer positive health effects. A sense of fulfillment and personal worth is achieved and changes in outlook and ability frequently result from the intergenerational experience. Above all, the interaction and commitment developed through multigenerational activities help form bonds of love and affection.

Intergenerational programs can be organized in different ways. Some successful arrangements include weekly meetings between a nursery school group and a senior citizen club, monthly visits to a nursing home by primary grade children for a party which includes specific activities in the recreation room, and shared holiday celebrations throughout the year for older adults and children at a community day care center. Whatever brings the age groups together, careful plans are necessary to create an atmosphere for joyful interaction.

The recreation coordinator or dance specialist will usually arrange and direct the sessions. Individual group leaders and class teachers should join in the planning and assist participants during the activity. To provide appropriate content and smooth interchanges, each group may be prepared separately before meeting together. Structured games and dances will be even more successful if taught and practiced in advance. The selection and progression of activities in each session involve consideration of the abilities of the participants. Pre-school and primary age children are usually very active with short attention spans. Independent older adults may be quite vigorous. Most residents and participants in nursing homes or day care centers, however, tire easily or are limited to sitting activities or fairly moderate movements. Therefore, resting

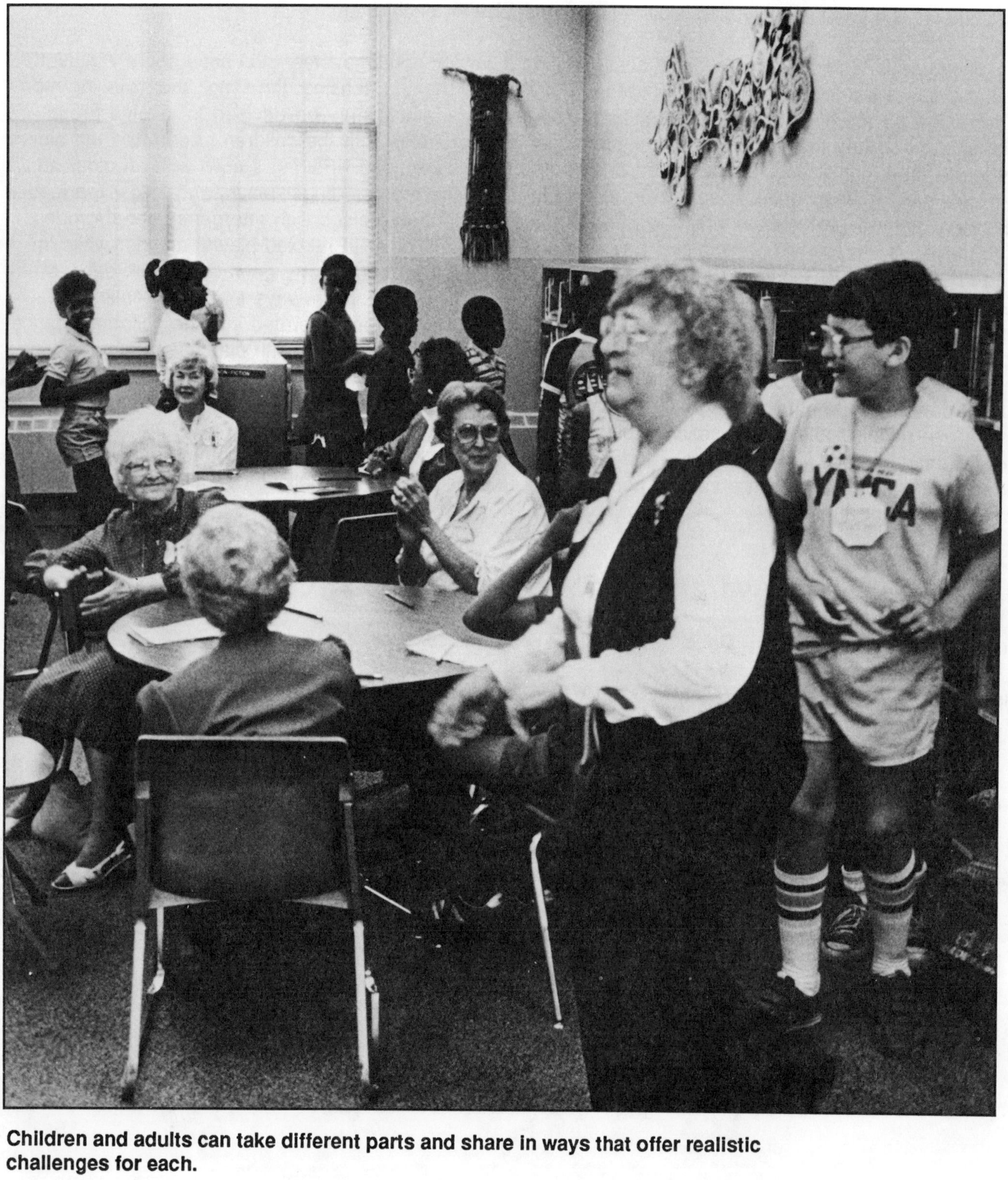

PHOTO COURTESY OF DAVID E. CORBIN

Children and adults can take different parts and share in ways that offer realistic challenges for each.

and thinking times, alternating singing and action games or two part dances that allow for "taking turns" can be scheduled. The sessions may also include time to perform for each other.

Sessions for combined age groups ideally include developmental movement to encourage a variety of energy and space use. Participants can engage in stretching, shaking, tensing, thrusting, and swinging motions for warm-up activities in various directional patterns. Variations may be devised to involve group members whether they are ambulatory or chairbound. Double circles with the children in one and the older adults in the other can accommodate varied energy and flexibility ranges. Pairing a child with an older adult may inspire greater effort and pleasure from the adult. Counting rhymes, finger plays, and follow the leader activities are all good vehicles in which to perform developmental exercises with intergenerational groups. Though these, young and old participants may sing and help each other in relaxed playful manner while improving spatial concepts, coordination, flexibility, and balance skills. Play-party games and folk dances encourage creativity. Children and adults can take different parts and share in ways that offer realistic challenges for each. More vigorous skipping, jumping, and running can be incorporated into the childrens' dance responses, while the adults will find expressive ways to join the dance pattern with clapping, stamping, and rocking phrases. Physical contact may often become a natural and enjoyable movement expression. Traditional folk dances in the ethnic background of the young and old group members may be performed with variations that use rhythm instruments, scarves, batons, and other props. In each instance, cooperative decision making, expanded movement responses, and joyful laughter usually result. These structured dance forms also provide opportunities to pass on a cultural heritage and emphasize the links between people in the continuum from the past to the future.

REFERENCES

Barlin, A. and Barlin, P. (1974). *Dance a folk song.* Los Angeles: Bowman Publishing Co.

Harris, J. A., Pittman, A.M. and Waller, M.S. (1978). *Dance awhile.* Minneapolis: Burgess Publishing Co.

Lindner, E.C., Harpaz, C.L., and Samberg, S. *Therapeutic dance/movement: Expressive activities for older adults.* New York: Human Sciences Press.

Lindner, E.C. and Harpaz, L. (1979). *Special dancing on you feet or in your seat.* Freeport, NY: Educational Activities, Inc.

Nelson, E. (1973). *Dancing games for children of all ages.* New York: Sterling Publishing Co.

Polk, E. (1972). *Orchestrated music for special children.* New York: Hoctor Records Co.

16

Dance Programs In Southeastern Connecticut

Pamela J. Lewis and Linda Deutch

Southeastern Connecticut currently boasts two innovative dance/fitness programs for the older adult population. Both of these programs are unique to this area and are called "Dance By the Sea" and "The Energy Hour". Before describing the individual programs, it may be helpful to note how they evolved in this shoreline community.

As an independent dance professional, educator, and performer, Pamela Lewis wanted to develop a dance/fitness program in the New London, Connecticut area. Due to the calming and healing qualities of the sea, the beach was chosen as an ideal location for a dance program. The city of New London was approached with the concept of "Dance By The Sea" and was pleased to sponsor the program.

Once the program began, it became apparent that there were many older adults attending the program who were not suited for the standard dance/fitness programs offered in the community. Many had suffered injuries and became disillusioned with the more hard-driving, fast-paced fitness programs. "Dance By the Sea" addressed this problem and was designed to target the special needs of the older adult population.

This led to the realization that if the needs of the people attending "Dance By the Sea" had been neglected, what about the remaining segment of the population who were isolated and did not have access to such a program? This question spurred a careful observation of various convalescent homes in the community. A needs assessment revealed that there were few dance/fitness programs taking place in convalescent homes. Most existing programs consisted of entertainment where people were merely passive observers and not active participants in the program. The remaining programs were too strenuous and were eventually discontinued. Hence "The Energy Hour" was established as a pilot program sponsored by the Adult Education Departments in the city of New London and the surrounding towns of Groton and Waterford.

Dance By the Sea

"Dance By the Sea" began in the summer of 1984. The program has received considerable attention from the local media and has attracted an increasing number of people over the years. The drop-out rate is low and approximately 75% of the current participants have been with the program since its inception. The age range is 30-88 years old and 98% are women. The program runs from July to September and consists of three morning classes, five days per week. Due to the success of "Dance By the Sea", the program has been expanded to include one morning class during the winter months. This class is held indoors near the beach.

"Dance By the Sea" reflects an integrated and holistic approach to dance and fitness. It proposes that dance and fitness do not simply involve the learning of techniques to be practiced and rehearsed. Rather, the underlying belief is that people must also have self-knowledge and body awareness before they can express themselves through movement. Therefore a major goal of "Dance By the Sea" is to educate people about this important relationship between the mind and body (Gelb, 1981; Donnelly, 1982).

In addition to the program's educational approach, "Dance By the Sea" participants have described the program as being therapeutic in nature. Ms. Lewis has generated this therapeutic quality by being open and perceptive to the needs of the people in each class. As a result of being with people on a daily basis and closely monitoring their needs, the class structure varies somewhat from day to day. As an individual, Ms. Lewis is also committed to self-improvement and shares this enthusiasm with her classes. People have reported this sharing of experience to be beneficial to add to a class spirit of well-being and growth.

Although there is some variation within classes, the "Dance By the Sea" program consists of four major components.

The first component and an integral part of the program is walking on the boardwalk. Walking is included for its aerobic benefits. It is also considered to be an appropriate form of exercise for the older adult because most people can walk regardless of their physical condition. Participants are encouraged to walk at their own pace and to calculate their time and distance.

Following a walk on the boardwalk is the Stretch/Strengthening portion of the program. This component is done on the sand and lasts for approximately 30 minutes. The purpose of the Stretch/ Strengthening component is to connect the mind and body through different postures and breathing. It is similar to yoga and is a blend of the Alexander (1984) technique and Kendall (1981) work on posture and body alignment. Many of the Stretch/Strengthening exercises are based on the principles of Alexander which teaches one how to use the body more efficiently. Kendall's work provided scientific knowledge of the various muscle groups. This knowledge was then implemented to teach people how to repattern different muscle groups, allowing them to move more effortlessly. In doing these exercises, people became aware of and learn to correct bad habits such as tension in the neck and shoulders, improper use of abdominal muscles, and poor body posture.

Dancing is the third component of the program. The dance component lasts approximately 20 minutes and takes place on the boardwalk under an open tent. The emphasis is on feeling alive and moving to music as opposed to learning dance steps and combinations. A wide variety of music is used and ranges from Bette Midler to Glenn Miller, African to Reggae and Rock N' Roll. The dance component is eclectic and is made up of diverse dance styles and techniques. Some of the movement is derived from modern Limon technique which includes lengthening and swinging motions to release tension in the shoulders and hips. Other dance forms are included which are reminiscent of a bygone era such as the Charleston and the Rhumba. Jazz dancing involving quick, sharp movements is also included in the

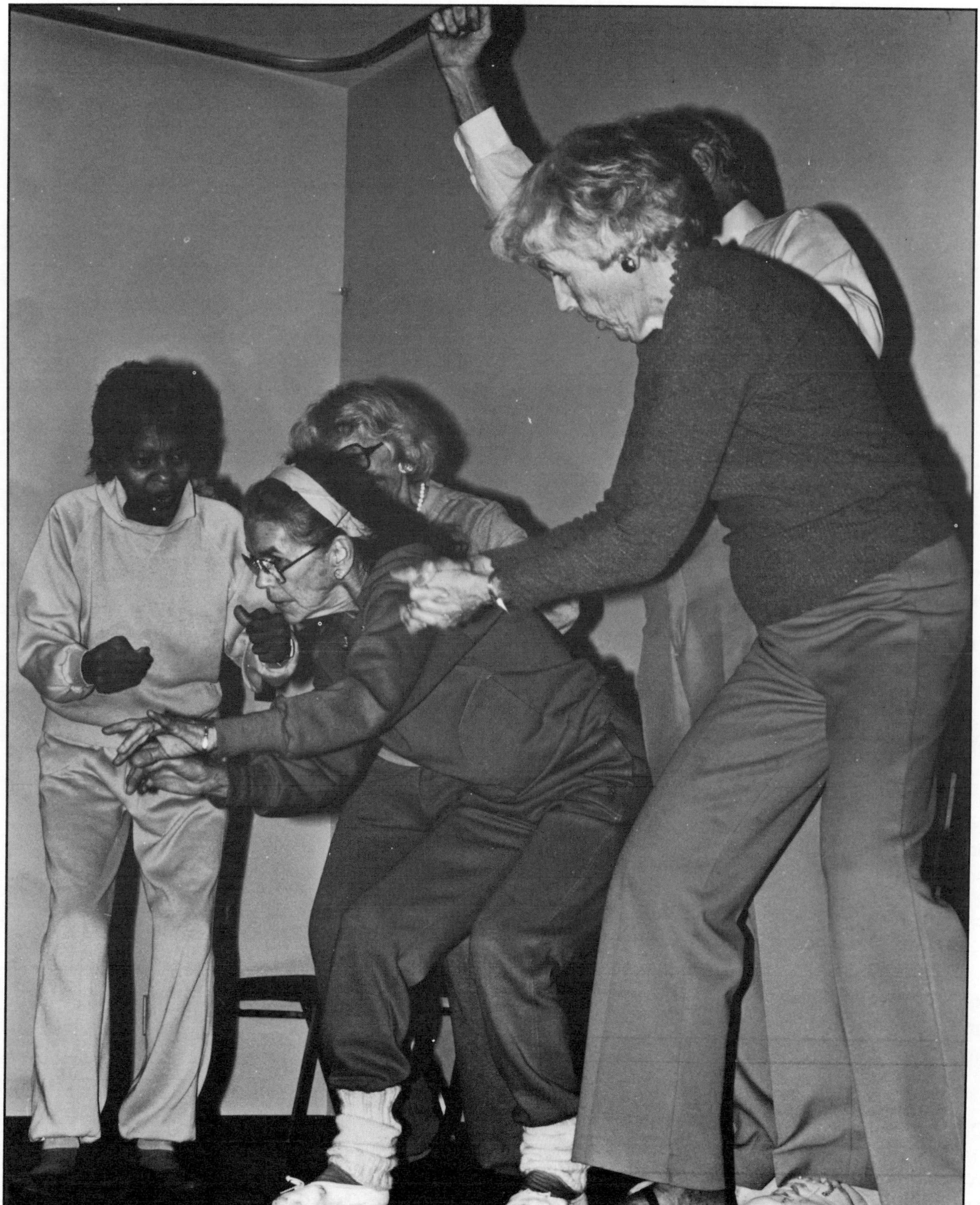

PHOTO COURTESY OF ANDRE RICHARDSON

A dance program can help to meet the basic, human needs of many older adults: physical contact, mental engagement, and social interaction.

repertoire as well as fitness dancing with its focus on muscle groups and strengthening. Ballet movements are used at the end as a means of slowing down and returning the body to its proper alignment.

The fourth and final portion of "Dance By the Sea" is Quiet Meditation on the beach which lasts 5-10 minutes. Meditation is done at the end of each class and leaves people feeling refreshed and ready to start the day. Breathing exercises and guided imagery are the techniques used for relaxation.

In addition to the above components, "Dance By the Sea" features guest teachers from other disciplines (e.g., Alexander, accupressure, massage, yoga). Outside teachers are reported to enhance the program and to broaden people's knowledge and experience of the body. This increased knowledge is then incorporated into the overall program. In each class, for example, people massage their feet and legs before dancing. This was learned from a Japanese teacher with expertise in yoga and aerobics.

In 1987, an evaluation of "Dance By the Sea" was conducted. The questionnaire was designed to assess whether people noticed any changes in their body awareness or general health as a result of the "Dance By the Sea" program. (The questionnaire is found at the back of the article). Many participants reported improvement with a health problem they had been experiencing. For instance, one person said the stiffness in her joints had been greatly relieved by "Dance By the Sea" classes. Another participant noted improvement with digestive problems as a result of learning better body posture (e.g., holding shoulders back and expanding the chest). "Dance By the Sea's" relaxation benefits were also noted to be helpful in stabilizing another participant's blood pressure.

Results of the questionnaire revealed that 95% of the participants noticed an improvement in body posture and overall body awareness. Most people also commented on "Dance By the Sea's" therapeutic benefits as well as it being a fun program.

The Energy Hour

"The Energy Hour" began in 1984. In the beginning, this program took place in three convalescent homes and has since been expanded to include 11 senior citizen facilities, one of which is an adult day care program.

As noted previously, in conducting the "Dance By the Sea" program, Ms. Lewis recognized the potential of adapting her program to the needs to a more isolated and older population. The first adaptation addressed this population's physical limitations. The program was redesigned with the exercises done in a sitting position making them less strenuous. The second adaptation was much more difficult. It involved overcoming participants' mental and social barriers resulting from institutionalization. For example, helplessness, passivity, and loneliness were observed in institutionalized participants.

It soon became clear that prior to teaching the benefits of dance and the mind/body connection, more basic human needs had to be addressed. These needs included physical contact, mental engagement, and a longing for social interaction with younger people. Movement and music became the medium for making this contact. The emphasis became wellness and the healing power of laughter and humor.

As with "Dance By the Sea", "The Energy Hour" can be broken down into four major components. During the first component, participants form a circle and touch each member of the class individually. Many people are surprised and delighted with this direct human contact. The second component, Warm-Up and Body Awareness, includes range-of-motion exercises. These are based on physical therapy exercises and are designed to loosen up joints and strengthen different muscles.

Following the warm-up, music is added for the third component. People learn simple dance movements that can be done sitting down. The music played has basic rhythm structures and ranges from waltzes and Glenn Miller to the Pointer Sisters. The routine often ends with a sign language dance done to the music "The Rose". This piece can be done with just the hands and many people find it touching and beautiful. Each person is danced with individually. Participants often say that they are grateful and happy to be asked to dance.

Reality Orientation is the fourth and final component. This portion of the program consists of games and exercises to stimulate the mind and to provide opportunities for self-expression. One game, for instance, is called "Pass the Cup of Knowledge". In this game, an empty cup is passed around a circle while music is being played. When the music stops, the person holding the cup is asked different questions. Depending on their level of ability and awareness, the person is asked certain autobiographical questions. Specific questions may be about family, friends or past accomplishments. The purpose of this game is to stimulate thinking and to show an interest in the person as an individual.

Another game consists of reading the "Dear Abby" column and inviting people to give their own advice. During this game, many people realize that they do indeed have something to give and that their opinion counts. This helps to combat feelings of worthlessness experienced by people who tend to be excluded from society. Humor is used throughout "The Energy Hour" which lends to an overall atmosphere of fun and well-being.

Conclusion

In conclusion, "Dance By the Sea" and "The Energy Hour" have demonstrated success with the older adult population. These programs show us that the needs of the older adult should not be neglected. They also support the underlying philosophy of adult education which proposes that it is never too late to learn, and that learning is a life-long process. Furthermore, due to the increasing growth of the older adult population, the success of these programs suggest that other communities could also benefit from programs of this type.

"Dance By the Sea" and "The Energy Hour" also have implications for physical and mental health. People in both programs have reported increased feelings of well-being in addition to improvement in their physical condition. Despite the growing health consciousness in this country, most approaches to dance and fitness aim for quick and immediate results. Although this holistic approach may take longer to learn, it is likely to have more long-term benefits. Learning proper body alignment, for instance, is something that one can carry with them and apply to many aspects of their life.

Murray Louis (1980) has said that "the body is an incredibly wise and knowledgeable source and knows a great deal more about the human experience than anyone could possibly learn in a lifetime." Perhaps this is best demonstrated by a 75 year old woman who was a participant of "The Energy Hour". This woman became ill, went into a coma, and could not speak. However, when familiar music was played by her bedside, she responded by moving her body from side to side. Our bodies may indeed remember longer than our brain. And they, like the old, have a wisdom that should be cherished.

Exercise by the Sea
Questionaire

name ______________________ date ______________________

age in years ______________________ days per week ______________________

1. As a result of taking this class, have you noticed any improvements with a health problem you may be experiencing? (arthritis, depression, colds, other)

2. Have you noticed any changes in the following? Explain briefly.

posture ______________________

abdominal strength ______________________

flexibility:
- spine ______________________
- neck ______________________
- leg and hip ______________________
- shoulder ______________________

total body awareness ______________________

dance coordination ______________________

ability to relax ______________________

diet ______________________

energy level ______________________

emotional self ______________________

relationship with:
- family members ______________________
- class members ______________________

self-esteem ______________________

sex life ______________________

overall health ______________________

other ______________________

3. A. What sections of the class have been *most beneficial* to you?

duet stretches ________
massage ________
chair warm-ups ________
dancing ________
the lie down ________
meditation ________
guest teachers ________

B. Your favorite section:

C. Your least favorite sections:

D. Comments about the class set-up and structure:

4. How could Pam improve her teaching and/or classes?

5. How would you compare this program to others you have taken in the past?

6. Other comments:

REFERENCES

Alexander, F.M. (1984). The use of the self. Long Beach, CA: Centerline.

Donnelly, J.E. (1982). Living anatomy. Champaign, IL: Human Kinetics.

Gelb, M. (1981). Body Learning: New York: Delilah Books.

Kendall, H.O., Kendall, F. P., and Beynton, D.A. (1981). Posture and pain. Malabar, FL: Robert E. Krieger.

Louis, M. (1980). Inside dance. New York: St. Martin.

17

Shared Movement Programs

College Students And Older Adults

Josie Metal-Corbin

At the University of Nebraska at Omaha, college students volunteer in an intergenerational project that regularly has brought dance to older adults over the past two years. Entitled "A Time to Dance," the project provides dance programs for older adults, trains volunteer personnel to establish dance programs, provides opportunities for generations to share experiences through dance, and demonstrates that dance is for everyone.

"A Time to Dance" is a cooperative effort between the university and the community. A dance educator serves as program director, brings together students from university dance classes and healthy older adults who participate in recreational programs offered by the Downtown Omaha Center for Seniors under the auspices of the Eastern Nebraska Office on Aging. Throughout the year sets of eight weekly dance classes are offered without charge to participants. The procedures used in establishing and implementing this program may serve as a model for other programs in intergenerational approaches to dance.

A visit to the Department of Parks and Recreation established the need for dance among older adults in the Omaha area, and resulted in a plan to include dance in the regular recreational programming for senior citizens. The pilot group included 20 university students, 25 older adults ranging in age from 55-85 years, and a dance educator from the University of Nebraska at Omaha.

Prior to the first class, an orientation session for university students acquainted them with class format and types of dance activities to be included in the program. The group discussed precautions for working with older adults and made a special effort to explain to university students that older adults are as heterogeneous a group as any other.

Students and older adults usually arrived 15 minutes early to socialize with each other. Music from the 20s, 30s and 40s served both as background to the conversation and as a stimulus for "life review." The music evoked many stories and memories that older adults shared with the younger generation. Armless, straight-backed chairs arranged around the space in a large circle enabled the leader to communicate visu-

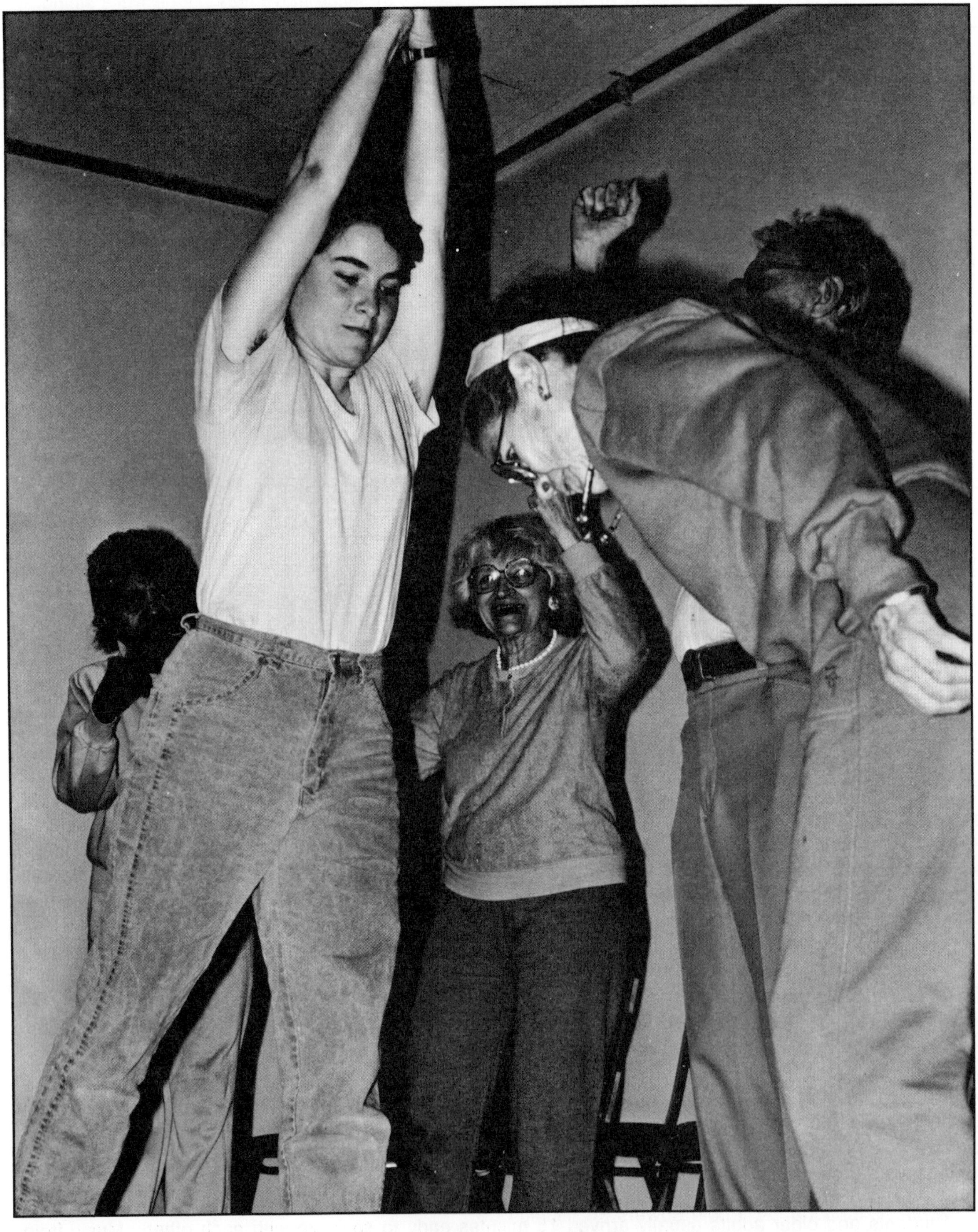

PHOTO COURTESY OF ANDRE RICHARDSON

"A Time to Dance" provides opportunities for college students and older adults to share the dance experience.

ally while acknowledging and encouraging participants. The movers were urged to recognize their own limitations and to self-monitor whenever appropriate. The emphasis was on comfort and safety while moving.

The class was comprised of a general warm-up, a sequence of dance movements done while sitting, standing, and locomoting, a special focus of the day, and cooling down activities. The first activity, a general warm-up, was done while participants were seated. Sometimes stretching bicycle innertubes was incorporated into this segment. These exercises, involving movement of major muscle groups, promoted flexibility, muscular strength, and endurance and increased blood circulation to the extremities. The adaptable bike innertubes can offer as great or as little resistance as each participant desires. Other warmups took the form of "Follow the Leader" using contracting and expanding movements of the arms, legs and torso. The general warm-up also included smooth jazz isolations.

Participants performed adaptations of dance steps and movements while seated. Some "dances" involved arm and hand patterns only, or leg and foot patterns only. Some were choreographed to allow some participants to remain seated while others stood and moved in front of the chairs. dance in the chairs was a way to accommodate participants' various health problems. It effectively accomplished one of the main goals of the project--to have *everyone* dance and share in the spirit of the dance. All of these dances were created by the dance educator and were based on traditional dance steps from tap, ballet, modern and jazz.

Line, circle, and partner dances, presented in the standing and moving activities segments, ranged from newly choreographed dances to familiar folk and social dances such as the Charleston, Tennessee Wig Walk, Hully Gully, Hora, and Hustle. Young and old participants were given time to present dances of their choice to the group. Whenever possible, the leader encouraged the group to sing along with the music.

The special focus or activity of the day ranged from large group work with a parachute to small group improvisation with poetry or props. The small groups provided time for socialization, cooperation, and shared creativity.

During the cooling down time relaxation activities, breathing exercises, and "dance in the chairs" could express a theme with sustained and flowing movement qualities.

New faces were present with each new session, but a core of students and older adults from the pilot program continue to return. The class format has evolved to include more elements of modern dance and improvisation. Tai Chi and Yoga have also been incorporated into the class as well.

Speaking on the meaning of life in old age, gerontologist Leo Missine stated " . . . .if younger people wish to have a meaningful later life, they must learn to respect, to like, and to love older people." The "Time to Dance" program is one means to that end.

REFERENCES

Caplow-Lindner, Harpaz, E.L. and Samberg, S. (1979). *Therapeutic dance movement: Expressive activities for older adults.* New York: Human Sciences Press.

Corbin, D.E. (1981). An exercise program for the elderly. *The Physical Educator.* 38(1): 46-49.

Corbin, D.E. (1981). *Psychological and physical aspects of self-perceived health status among older adults.* Unpublished doctoral dissertation. University of Pittsburgh.

Corbin, D.E. & Metal-Corbin, J. (1983). *Reach for it: A handbook of exercise and dance activities for older adults.* Dubuque, IA: Eddie Bowers Publishing Co.

Leviton, D., and Santoro, L. (Eds.). (1980). *Health, physical education, recreation and dance for the older adult: A modular approach.* Reston, VA: AAHPERD.

V. Intergenerational Dance

18

Dance Belongs To Everyone

Jeff Bliss

How often do you dance? Every day, once a month, only when you have a room to yourself? When you are lost in the crowd? The urge to move, to dance, is the urging of life itself, though many of us withhold that reaction when the opportunity arises. What stops us from moving, from dancing? The most common answer you will hear is "I can't dance". The answer is based on a common perception in today's specialized society, a dancer is someone who has the technical ability to do things with their bodies that we can not do. An intergenerational modern dance company, the Dancers of the Third Age, from Washington, D.C., is working to change that perception.

Founded in 1975 by Liz Lerman, the Dancers of the Third Age (DTA) is comprised of senior adults between the ages of 60 and 90 along with members of The Dance Exchange, Ms. Lerman's professional company. Though some of the DTA members joined the group with no previous performance experience, they have become seasoned performers over the years. Their audiences range from elementary schools to universities, art galleries, senior centers, national conventions, and festivals across the United States and in Europe. Their message is quite clear, "Everyone can dance."

As noted in the Washington Weekly "one glimpse of their art and one bids farewell to the notion that dance -- and life for that matter -- should be restricted to 21 year old slyphs." And from the Philadelphia magazine, After Dark, it was reported that "in the presence of our elders, I felt exalted."

The performances include demonstrations of a typical senior class format and then moves on to improvised and set pieces that have been choreographed by the group's founder Liz Lerman and its director, Don Zuckerman. Throughout the performance the audience is drawn into participation in the process of making dances, they become the dancers they have come to watch. This approach is just as exciting for the DTA members as it is for the audience. As Jess Rea, a veteran member of the troupe notes, "When the body moves, the spirit moves." And move they do. At a recent performance at D.C. Village, an innovative long-term care facility run by the city of Washington, all types and sizes of people joined the Company in an improvisational dance. Young people and older adults: some standing, some in wheelchairs, and others with canes were strutting, scooping, and turning across the floor together. To watch and participate in such an activity is a joyous experience, the kind of experience that

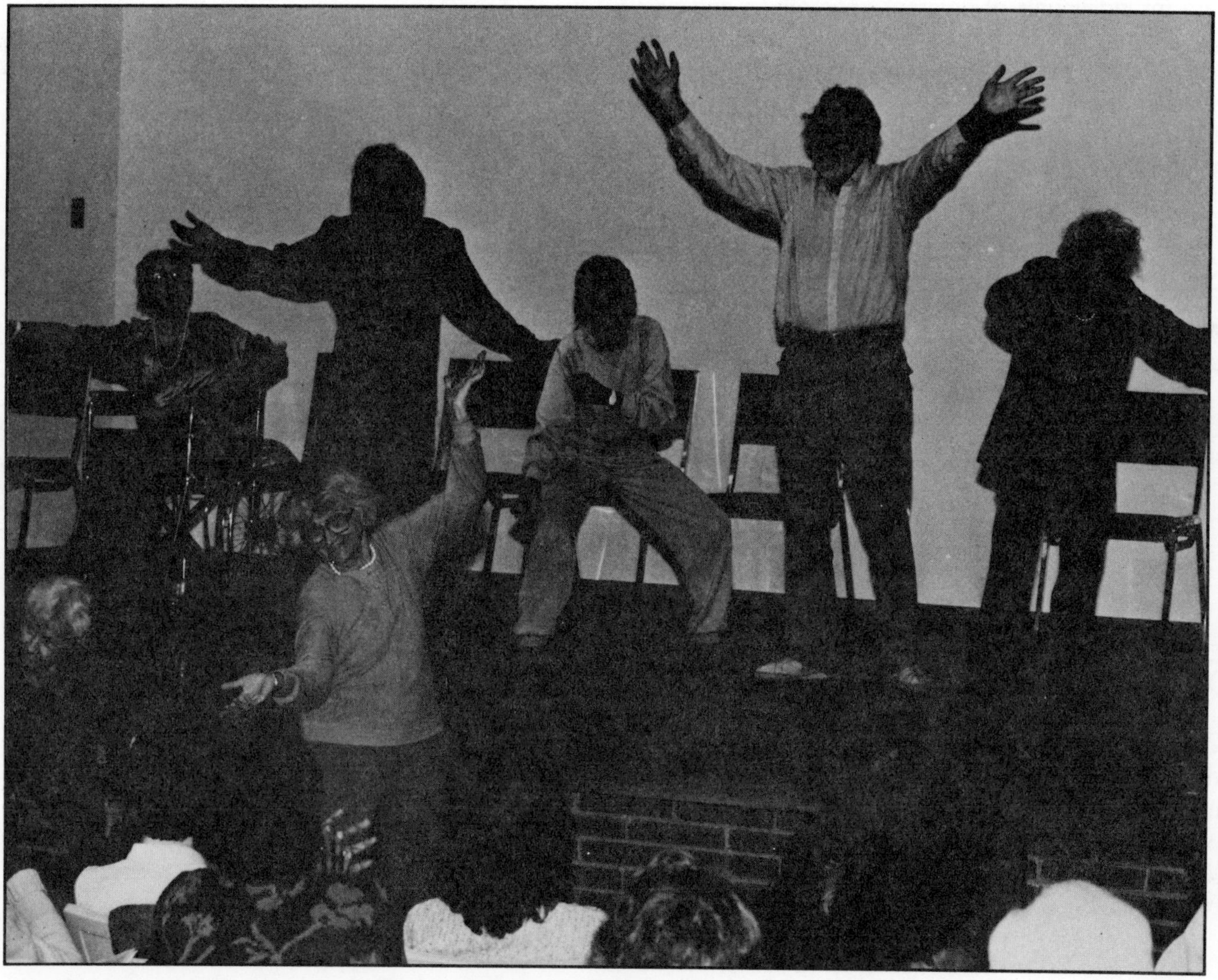

PHOTO COURTESY OF ANDRE RICHARDSON

The Dancers of the Third Age is comprised of senior adults between the ages of 60 and 90. Their message is clear: "Everyone can dance."

can change people's definition of themselves as dancers. Today the opportunities to dance together are rare for individuals of different generations and backgrounds. The Dancers of the Third Age are creating the climate for the opportunities to flourish across the country; Liz Lerman's vision is becoming a reality. As she notes in her book, Teaching Dance to Senior Adults, "This work with older adults has convinced me of things about dance that I suspected all along.... Dancing, with its expressive and creative aspects, is a natural activity for all human beings.... the inherent characteristics and benefits of dance belong to everyone."

19

An Interview With Liz Lerman

Cynthia P. Ensign

Liz Lerman is director of the Dance Exchange in Washington, D.C. This interview, conducted by Cynthia P. Ensign, focuses on her senior adult performing group, Dancers of the Third Age.

Cynthia P. Ensign: With whom do you work -- what kinds of people, what ages?

Liz Lerman: Through the Dance Exchange I actually work with many kinds of people and with a wide age span. Dancers of the Third Age refers specifically to my performing group of senior adults. They range in age from 60 to 88. All are independent enough to be able to come to rehearsals once a week and to perform approximately once a week. Some do need to be picked up, and one is in a wheelchair.

Dancers of the Third Age is only part of my work with the senior adult. I also teach classes in the community--in nursing homes and in senior activity centers.

CPE: How are the dancers for the Dancers of the Third Age selected?

LL: Sometimes after viewing a performance some will call and want to get involved. At other times I have invited some members of my classes to join. No one has ever been turned away. Usually they self-select according to their interest and commitment to the performing group.

I use some of the dancers from the Third Age in my choreography for my younger, professional company. For this choreography I select the seniors to perform. I've tried to use many different dancers from the Third Age.

CPE: How did you get started working with dance for the senior adult?

LL: I've always felt that dance belongs to everybody. I've felt that working with seniors--with what they can contribute to and what they can gain from dance--has been missing in the professional dance world.

The catalyst that brought about my work in dance and with the senior adult was my mother's death. I wanted to do a piece about my family just before her death and needed older people as part of the dance. To find people for the dance I began teaching classes in the local community. From these classes I asked for volunteers. And

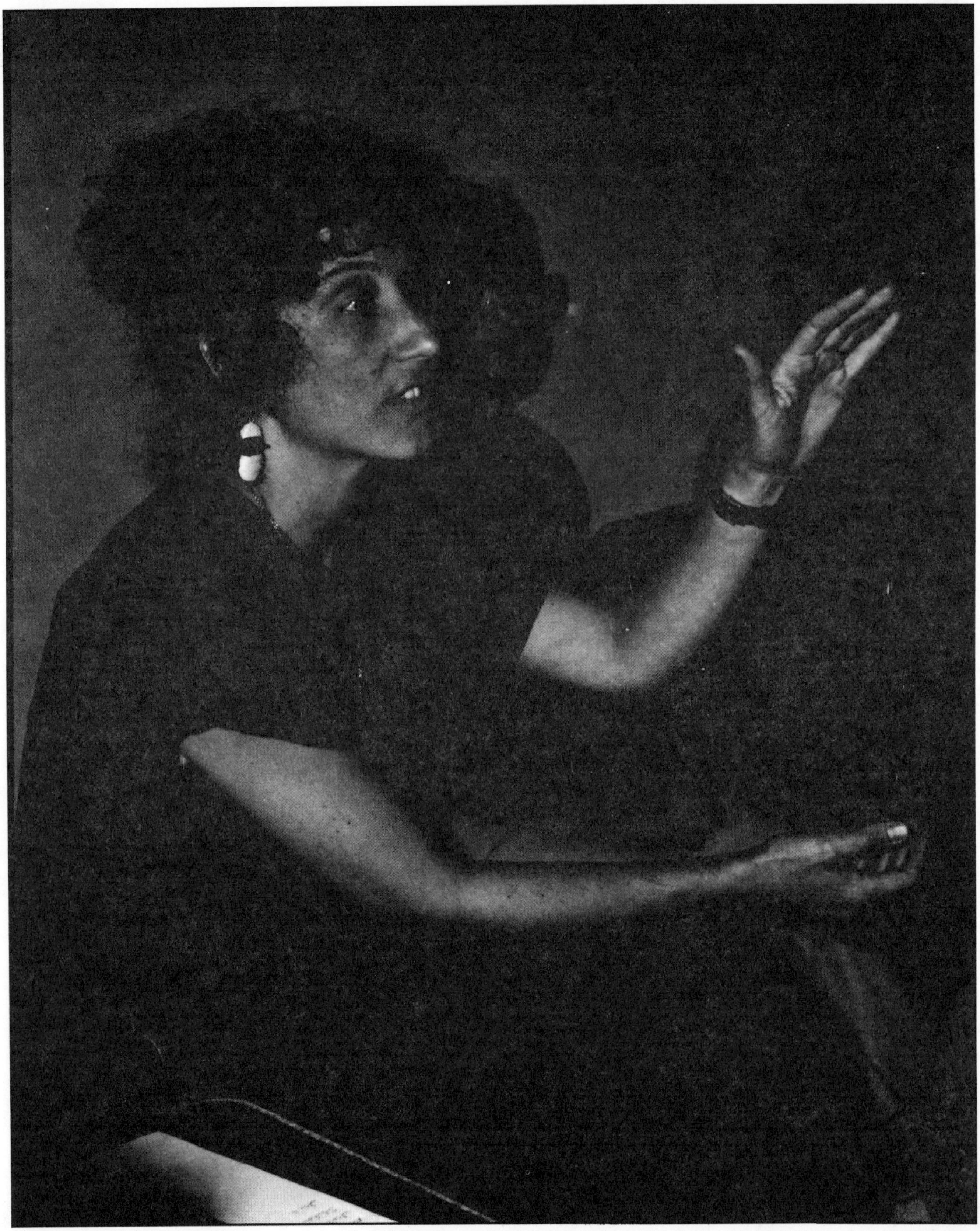

PHOTO COURTESY OF ANDRE RICHARDSON

Liz Lerman is Director of the Dance Exchange in Washington, D.C.

from that point in 1975 I've continued to teach classes for the senior adult and drawn upon them for dancers of the Third Age. Now my choreography for my professional company often requires older dancers. I feel that my present work with the senior adult has had a very organic evolvement.

CPE: How have you been able to bring people with little or no background in dance or movement, and perhaps with even negative experiences in these areas, to the point where they feel comfortable enough to perform?

LL: I guess it gets down to what I view as beautiful on stage. I prefer honesty in movement over technical ability--no matter who the dancer. I like to see human beings moving with movement that is inherently true to them. Also, how the dancers are treated, how they are supported is important. That helps them to feel comfortable with dance and movement and performing in front of others. In rehearsals we move from dance exercises to structured improvisations and from there select the movement material.

Our [Third Age] performances are quite informal. Much of each performance is structured improvisation and each usually involves some audience participation. The dancers don't wear costumes.

In my own choreography, however, in which I have specifically selected the senior dancers, the seniors do wear costumes; they must learn specific cues; they must stay up for rehearsals; and they are subject to criticism in the press.

CPE: How are dancers for Dancers of the Third Age choreographed?

LL: Both the dancers and I take turns. Sometimes it is their turn and other members of the company help them shape their ideas. Some of the dancers have even begun their own choreography separate from their work with me. At other times it is my turn. Usually I find my turn with choreography for my younger, professional company when I select dancers from the Third Age to perform with them. But I also use ideas that have originated with the Third Age group for my younger company. When I do so, I consult with my Third Age dancers.

CPE: What, to you, are some of the values of dance performance?

LL: I feel performance is a natural state. It's part of everybody. We don't feel comfortable with performance because of the way we're taught to think of it. I include some performance within each class I teach. It's usually at the end. I'll divide the class in half and each half will watch the other half. I feel there is a sense of purpose to be gained from performing. I feel that if someone has something to say or express--not something imposed on them--that the experience of performing will be meaningful.

The relationship that has developed between dance and the local community because of the Dancers of the Third Age has been remarkable. I think the mix of the dancers who go back to the rest of their lives in the community is important. And correspondingly what they bring to dance from their many perspectives can make dance all the richer.

20

Teaching Dance To Senior Adults

Liz Lerman

I am a dancer. I teach, choreograph, and perform. These facts affect the way I experience the episodes in my life. Seven years ago, my mother died of cancer. While she was sick, we spent hours together talking of our lives. During these conversations, my mind raced with provocative stage images of dancers moving in and out of her landscape. I always imagined older bodies as part of the scene, usually representing long-lost relatives, or I saw pictures of my mother's own body floating Chagall-like through the living room.

After her death, I returned to my home in Washington, D.C., and began to look for older people to fill the needs of this developing dance, and that is what led me to teach dance classes at The Roosevelt for Senior Citizens. I already had experience in working with unconventional dancers, that is to say, people not highly trained but very willing to move, learn, and express with their bodies. By this time in my life, I knew how to find such performers. I would go to a group that already existed for some other purpose and teach modern dance classes, and when a safe emotional environment had been established, I would ask for volunteers to be in a dance.

That is what I did, and after six months of classes, the dance *Woman of the Clear Vision* was premiered. Making that dance reminded me that performance is a wonderful process for building community among people who would not otherwise find themselves together. In this case, while confronting issues about life and death, young people and old people were also able to rehearse and grow as artists, to learn to be comfortable in each other's environment, and to pay attention to each other's lives.

This work with older adults has convinced me of things about dance that I suspected all along -- things I knew as a child dancing and things I came to know later as a questioning professional dancer. Dancing, with its expressive and creative aspects, is a natural activity for all human beings. Although the beautifully developed ability of the professional dancer makes for a spectacular display of human potential, it is also true that the inherent characteristics and benefits of dance belong to everyone.

This chapter is reprinted with permission from *Teaching Dance to Senior Adults* (Preface) by Liz Lerman, 1984. Courtesy of Charles C. Thomas, Publisher, Springfield, Illinois.

Dance magically combines exercise, self-expression, fun group activity, intellectual stimulation, and spiritual uplift. All people should have access to these activities no matter what their age, ability, or body type.

This work clearly has value for the participants, but it is also important as a symbol of the values a society incorporates for its culture. If art reflects life, certainly it is no surprise to see contemporary dancers pushing for technical virtuosity, for if there is a symbol for our age it must be technology. Dancing artisits are no different from anyone else in their urge to achieve efficiency and perfection.

Unfortunately, this places enormous pressure on the development of the technical aspect of dance. There are, however, many other facets of dance to discover, maintain, and develop. They include expressiveness, the exploration of contemporary themes, and the affirmation of a community's deeply felt ties. Older dancers can contribute in these areas.

Senior adults, particularly those who begin studying dance after age sixty, will probably not become fine technical dancers. What they bring to the activity , however, whether it is class warm-ups, improvisation, or informal performing, is an expressive body filled with life experiences. They remind us not only that dance belongs to everyone but that it can speak on many different levels. To ask a senior adult to do a fast, repeatable combination of ballet steps, for example, will mock both the person and the movement itself. But, when the person moves in harmony with an idea or emotion, with a movement vocabulary that is inherently personal in the body, the result is sometimes staggeringly beautiful.

People feel better when they dance. People learn about themselves and their world when they dance. People recognize their limits, strive to overcome them, and can see the results when they dance. These things occur as a person trains to dance. The goal is to develop a person at home in his or her body, a person capable of expressing feelings and ideas through movement, unafraid to move freely in a room filled with people, capable of learning a sequence or structure, willing to try new things, and willing to engage in the simple act of moving for no reason beyond the joy of the experience.

As I have travelled and worked this last decade, I have taught over 3000 dance classes. Everywhere I go I see vast numbers of dancers being trained for a world where no one will pay them to do what they so love to do. The demands of the field wear heavily on many people, clearly emphasizing a narrow definition of dance as a performance art. In the end, for many, the pressures are too great, and they choose to leave dance. With that decision they lose a major part of their lives simply because they did not fit into a precise and rigid structure.

It is hoped that the theory behind the teaching in this book can help younger dancers see that there are alternatives, not just in terms of social rewards and fulfillment as one experiences the joy that dancing can bring to older people but also in the effects this work can has on the dancer herself, as a dancer. There are people to be taught, people who will want to see their dances, people who will want to dance with them. This is in no way compromising to their art, their technique, or their own performing aspirations. It is broadening for everyone.

The significance of this work lies ultimately in its ability to bridge the isolation of artists and that of the elderly. The validation and meaning come from positive use of mind and body, the sharing of knowledge, and the resultant joy of people dancing together.

21

All My Grandmothers Could Sing

An Interdisciplinary And Intergenerational Choreography

Josie Metal-Corbin And Roger E. Foltz

"All My Grandmothers Could Sing" was an intergenerational, choreographic work that integrated original dance, music, videography, costume, and scenic design with poetry. During the 1984-85 academic year, faculty members and students from five different departments within the University of Nebraska at Omaha (UNO), performers from the Omaha community, and poets from across the state of Nebraska collaborated to create original choreography and music. The work incorporated three generations of dancers interpreting selected poems from a collection of poetry, *All My Grandmothers Could Sing*, by Nebraskan women.

Faculty members on a university urban-commuting campus, such as the University of Nebraska at Omaha, tend to work in isolation. They do not reach out to connect with other disciplines. The interdepartmental cooperation that flowered in "All My Grandmothers Could Sing" began with a similar 1983-84 work, "Au Jardin Zoologique," which integrated dance, music, video, and the environment of the Henry Doorly Zoo of Omaha. This zoo project was composer W. Kenton Bales and choreographer Josie Metal-Corbin's first venture into dance and original music for video, and only the second videodance project for videographer Bill Scollon. As a result of this first collaborative effort, we devised a checklist for future interdisciplinary work, and as "All My Grandmothers Could Sing" began to evolve, these guidelines proved to be quite helpful.

1. Involve all directors and artistic personnel during the conceptual phases of the project.
2. Discuss each collaborator's expectations for the final product.
3. Gain a working knowledge of each other's discipline. Become acquainted with the language of each area.
4. Plot a timetable immediately to allow time for the creative process, the rehearsals, the videotaping, and the postproduction phases.

5. Acquaint dancers, musicians, technicians, and video crew with all facets of the project so that they can handle the inevitable changes and artistic compromises that occur in a collaborative work.
6. Expect the unexpected. Be organized, be prepared, but above all be flexible.

The interdisciplinary and intergenerational work, "All My Grandmothers Could Sing," included the authors, Carol Petersen (poet, College of Business Administration), Janet Sussman (costume designer, Dramatic Arts), Denise Brady (poetry typesetting, Fine Arts Press), Michael Brooks (scenic designer, Dramatic Arts), as well as off-campus member Bill Scollon (videographer, KETV Television). This work was premiered at the University's Spring Dance Concert by "The Moving Company," a performing modern dance troupe for students under the auspices of the School of Health, Physical Education, and Recreation. In addition to three performances at "The Moving Company" concert, a videotape of the work opened the Senior Citizen Celebration Days, cosponsored by UNO's Gerontology Program and the Eastern Nebraska Office on Aging.

Integration of poetry

Creating a work reflecting Nebraska or the Great Plains region was a decision made during the project's developmental phase. Shortly thereafter the choreographer discovered a recently published collection of poems by Nebraskan women, *All My Grandmothers Could Sing*. Edited by Judith Sornberger (1983), the poetry collection captures Nebraskan women's experiences from pioneer days to present.

Integrating dance with this poetry required that the choreography be structured to harmonize with the meaning of the poetry so that the observer would not be confused by conflicting stimuli.

Elizabeth Hayes cites three approaches to a collaboration of this nature. (1) The words may preface the choreographic work, setting the mood or stating the purpose of the dance. (2) The spoken word may be incorporated within the dance by having the dancers speak the words or by having a choral group or reader read the poetry. (3) Words and the dance may be presented simultaneously or alternately. This project sought to enhance both dance and poetry without sacrificing the artistic independence of either one.

Before proceeding with the project, we sought permission to use the poems from both the publisher and the individual poets. Permission was needed not only for reading the poems during the live performance, but also for the videotape and for a special commemorative printing of the poetry by the University's Fine Arts Press.

Work with the composer

Having made the decision to connect dance to a series of poems, the choreographer's next step was to decide on the music for the piece. Often, a choreographer chooses to use existing music, as it is easier simply to seek out pieces that suggest the mood of the work and then tape those selections. The choreographer may then address other aesthetic and technical aspects of the project. In this instance, however, the choreographer believed that the vivid poetic imagery required original music to capture the special moods evoked by each poem.

At this point the authors, having agreed to the possibility of a collaboration, studied the poetry individually, reconvening later to exchange ideas on the project's potential. The following improvisational session, in which the authors experimented with various musical ideas and movement phrases, proved to be a harmonious way to work out compromises in the creative process. Thus they were able to commit themselves to biweekly meetings five months before the premiere of the work to assure that they shared a common vision for each poem, that the music suggested movement conducive to dance, and to assure that the tempos and timings were possible for the dancers. Subsequent sessions enhanced the spirit of collaboration between the choreographer and composer. Planning and agreeing upon methods of work in advance prevented last minute dance and score alterations which often take place during the stress of the final rehearsal week.

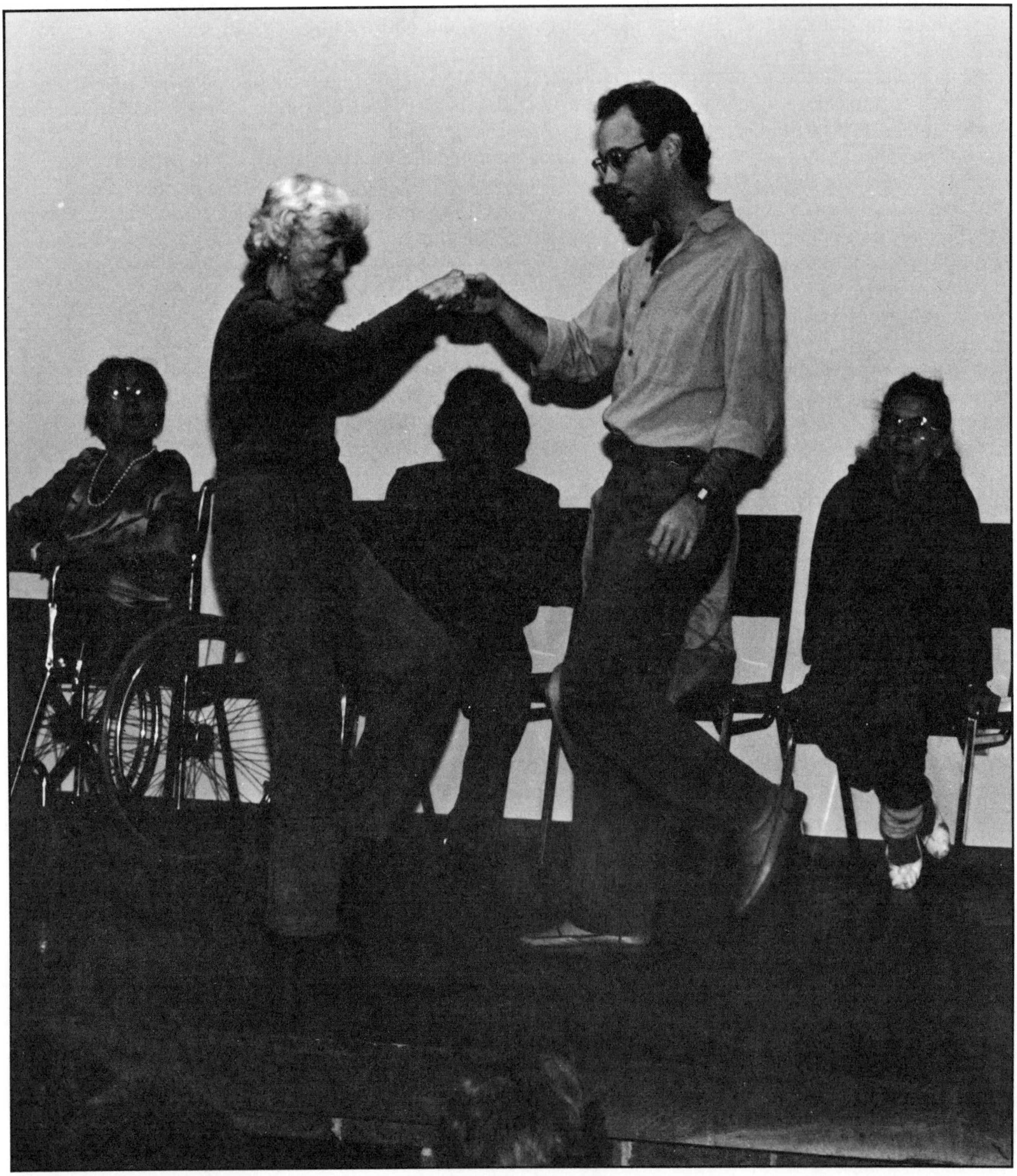

PHOTO COURTESY OF ANDRE RICHARDSON

The intergenerational choreography provided an opportunity for participants to view one another as individuals rather than in age-defined categories of "under 30" and "over 65."

Funding

As the project began to unfold, it became apparent that funding would need to be addressed. Since "The Moving Company" operates on a modest budget, funding was sought from several sources within the university, and from the Omaha community and the state. Funding was granted from the University Committee on Research for a videographer, a music copyist, a photographer, a costume construction supervisor, and a scenic crew member. The Committee also financed costume fabric, music copying supplies, fine arts press printing supplies, scenic construction materials and production expenses for a professional sound recording of the musical score.

Services ranging from secretarial support to faculty involvement came from the School of Health, Physical Education and Recreation; Department of Music; Department of Dramatic Arts; University Television; and the Fine Arts Press. The College of Fine Arts supported honoraria for the performing musicians and UNO's Gerontology Program assisted with the videotaping. The Nebraska Arts Council awarded a mini-grant to fund the composer's work.

The project's patchwork funding called for a mound of paperwork by the choreographer and composer. The process, however frustrating, promoted the project by bringing it to the attention of more people. These efforts uncovered additional ideas, in-kind services, and other avenues of financial support.

Intergenerational performers

Although American society does not hold high expectations for the older performer, three generations of performers ranging in age from 18 to 83 years translated their experience and the wisdom of the aged into a vibrant, creative work.

Choreography for the concert stage, traditionally designed to exhibit professionally trained dancers, should not be limited to the few elite performers. The creative and expressive powers of modern dance can provide an environment through which people of all ages can probe memories and present feelings. As Missinne and Lorenzen (1982) have observed, although older people suffer decreasing strength, energy level, and sensory power, they bring the gift of accumulated experience and knowledge of the world and of themselves to a work of art. "Potentially, they have the most to say about what it means to be human." While older people may engage in recreational folk, social, square or ballroom dance, only a few programs include them in a formal performance.

Observers have noted that choreographers and audiences giving unprecedented emphasis to the competitive aspect of dance, are demanding more technical virtuosity from performers. The focus on the dancer as a technician reflects a narrow view of dance art and affords to only a few the privilege of performing. "All My Grandmothers Could Sing" took a broader view of dance. It attempted to discover the technical as well as expressive movement potential of the older dancer and to develop choreography that did not compromise the art, but rather expanded the scope of performance. By choreographic design, this project used gestures and natural movements of older adult performers as a basis for parts of the choreographic structure and development.

The intergenerational choreography provided both the performers and the audience an opportunity to view one another as individuals, rather than in age-defined categories of "under 30" or "over 65." It created an environment suitable for observing, discovering, and appreciating the special contributions of each age to the project.

Videotape production

As planning for "All My Grandmothers Could Sing" progressed, the videographer began to attend rehearsals and to design the videotape which was shot during the final rehearsal week. The special qualities of the video -- close-ups, juxtapostions of images, and slow motion -- enabled the videographer to experiment with a new perspective on the dance. Follow shots, posterization, and other video digital effects were integrated into the final editing.

To prepare for the video production, the composer conducted a recording at a professional studio with the flutist, clarinetist, harpist, and pianist. This tape provided not only the soundtrack for the videotape but also an accurate musical score at technical rehearsals until musicians were incorporated into the work.

Because the budget permitted only two rehearsals with the musicians, the dancers and musicians did not perform together until the final dress rehearsal. Fortunately the dancers had to adjust only to minor tempo alterations.

Often dancers do not have the luxury of working in finished costumes and with a completed set before technical rehearsals. Advance planning minimized these last minute complications, as the costume designer and the scenic and lighting designer had spent time with the choreographer during the conceptual stages of the work. The poetry also was inserted during this technical week. The transitions from poetry to dance to poetry throughout the work were critical to keep the piece connected and flowing. A distinguished area actress from the Omaha Community Playhouse, with fifty years of acting experience, incorporated the poetry easily into the total work.

Learning collaboratively

The authors' experience with other artistic projects taught them that creators of art are not necessarily the most objective evaluators of their own efforts. Thus they were persuaded that outside evaluators should be secured to analyze the overall artistic merit of the project. But just as the creators of the art work are not always reliable critics, neither are friends and colleagues. The choreographer and composer therefore asked representatives from the arts community to evaluate the concert performance of "All My Grandmothers Could Sing." The critics used adjudication criteria forms adapted from one developed by the Educational Testing Service and used by the dance component of the National Arts Award in 1980.

On a 1 to 5 scale (5 is highest achievement), the panel gave the production 4.75. They agreed that the many facets of the production came together as a single artistic statement. They suggested further "tightening," and some of their ideas were incorporated in the videotape editing and postproduction.

Over 600 people viewed "The Moving Company" performances and about 250 saw the videotape at the Senior Citizens' Celebration Days. Broadcast twice on "Omaha Weekly," a magazine show on the university's educational channel, and cablecast three times during the summer and fall of 1985 on the local cable channel, the tape helped increase the number of individuals able to experience "All My Grandmothers Could Sing" to an estimated 30,000. In a metropolitan area of under 500,000 an audience of 30,000 is significant for an artistic event such as this.

Performers indicated that "All My Grandmothers Could Sing" was a success on another dimension, bringing together 30 individuals, many of whom did not know one another. This endeavor stimulated a deeper understanding of other arts disciplines while gaining a respect for the older performer.

The meetings, time, funding, and frustrations all take a heavy toll in such an undertaking, but the benefits of throwing oneself into areas previously not visited is rewarding and enriching. Both the intergenerational and interdisciplinary aspects of the experience enable one to develop not only new understandings of other arts and other generations, but to gain new insights into self and art.

REFERENCES

Hayes, E. (1955). *Dance Composition and Production.* New York, NY: The Ronald Press.

Lerman, L. (1984). *Teaching dance to senior adults.* Springfield, IL; Charles C. Thomas.

Missinne, L. and Lorenzen, L. (1982). The new 'wonder drug.' *Perspective on Aging,* 11(3), 15.

This project was funded in part by the Nebraska Arts Council and the University of Nebraska at Omaha Committee on Research, College of Education, College of Fine Arts, School of Health, Physical Education and Recreation, and Gerontology Program.

22

Dance for Older Adults in a Worship Setting

Doug Adams

In a growing number of worship settings where dance is welcomed regularly, dancers and movement educators are involving older adults in the sharing and creation of dances that help them experience and express their faith. Because movement and touch continue to communicate long after other modes of communication decline, dance may involve older adults and persons with handicaps to a much more profound level than other forms of expression. Hymns, carols, chants, and prayers familiar to the participants may provide a rhythmic structure to which movement may be added, just as gestures added to phrases of a hymn give new meaning to the words.

The participants themselves can be called upon to translate the words into movement by inventing and adding movements that carry meanings for them. Older adults may substitute blinking their eyes in hymns of joy which suggest a leap into the air. Leaping in the air is an unsettling, disorienting, surprising activity, and the older adults may find that blinking helps them experience some of these same unsettling and surprising qualities.

Movement ideas that have worked successfully with older adults in worship and home/nursing settings where dance was made a participatory activity are described here.

Hand holding and other hand touching contacts are particularly effective additions to movement. Holding hands is a vital activity for many people, and is one of the most powerful links with reality for those whose other senses are failing. Touching, stroking, and holding hands should be maximized at every opportunity. The participants may indicate the underlying beat by squeezing held hands to changing rhythms, an action both invigorating and community building.

Bowing and leaning activities may substitute for other movement ideas for chairbound participants. The head and neck may be involved in all sorts of bowing activity. Leaning forward in wheelchairs (or simply tilting heads forward) can successfully substitute for dancing into the cirlce's center. Leaning torso or heads to the left and right substitute for walking or running in those directions. Where neck problems restrict torso or head movements, the older adults suggest substituting tongue movements.

Suggested movement patterns may call for the raising of arms and the raising of joined hands. Facilitating arm raising will help motivate all participants to attempt the movement even if they can move their arms only a few inches above their laps. The arms may also be swung together in an arc as if the adults were walking along the street. Even simple arm raising movements provide a muscular workout in an movement session.

Use of the eyes in contact with others can evoke many feelings of belonging and being involved with other movers. Eye movements may suggest other movements or feelings. For example, blinking may demonstrate moments of rejoicing or surprise. Older adults have said that the blinking of their eyes allows them to break up mind sets and to give them a fresh perspective.

Percussive movements such as stomping feet, snapping fingers, and clapping hands provide an easy way to participate in beat keeping. The leader should suggest several methods of accomplishing this task to allow for various handicaps or disabilities.

In combining movement with hymns and carols, a circle formation has been used very successfully. One or two concentric circles work well when there is a large number of participants. It allows people to see, even to touch, other people in front of, behind, and to the side of themselves.

These movement ideas may be easily recombined for use with many hymn and carol patterns. The movement leader has only to reflect for a moment to find many additional movements. After one worship service that involved many older adults with various handicaps, a student noted that these adults became most alert and involved when the arts were used, and when hand contacts were made among them. The student commented that she herself was most alert at these significant times. The older adults' response underscored her own experience and focused on what are the most important parts of the worship for all persons--moments of physical expression and personal contact.

REFERENCES

Adams, Doug. *Dancing Christmas carols.* The Sharing Company, P.O. Box 2224, Austin, TX 78767.

Blessin, Ann Marie. *Sacred dance with the physically and mentally handicapped.* The Sharing Company, P.O. Box 2224, Austin, TX 78767.

Riordan, Anne (Ed). (1980). *Dance for the handicapped.* Reston, VA: AAHPERD.

23

A Moving Experience: Young Children and Older Adults

Intergenerational Dance Under 6 and Over 60

Erna Caplow Lindner and Leah Harpaz

Creative dance experiences can bridge the gap between generations. As our society looks favorably on extended families and shared resources, we are finding more opportunities to bring young people and elders together. The age separations caused by geography and social organizations are not being reversed. Many community centers, schools, houses of worship, nursing homes, and residences are realizing that varied age groups can share space and staff members. The resulting programs offer the advantages of both enriched content and economic efficiency. Non-verbal, spontaneous rhythmic movement activities are ideal for intergenerational communication.

Young and old participants in shared movement programs may reap different benefits. For the older generation, contacts with children often produce immediate responses of delight and rekindled interest in the present and the future. The shared activities are eagerly anticipated and the raised energy levels and increased physical participation attest to the positive effects. A sense of fulfillment and personal worth is achieved. Often a spontaneous change of outlook and ability results from intergenerational experiences. For example, there have been numerous instances when an elderly person temporarily put down a cane and took a youngster's hand to join the dancing circle. Smiles and songs sometimes replaced the vacant stares of withdrawn individuals.

Groups with mixed age participants offer the children extra one-to-one attention, non-judgemental acceptance, and patient assistance which may not be available in their home or school environments. Traditional movement activities will be passed on to them and different cultures can be shared so that a heritage is maintained. Even historical information may be included through the reminiscences of the older group members. The youngsters may also develop more positive views of aging through the role models of the elders.

Both old and young will enjoy sharing rhymes and games. "Miss Piggy" and "Miss Muffett", "Spider Man" and "Humpty Dumpty" can be joyfully exchanged to create respect for each generation's experiences. Above all, the interaction and commitment developed through multi-generational activities help form bonds of love and affection.

Program Organization

Programs for young children and older adults can be organized in various ways. Some arrangements that have been successful include: weekly sessions in which a nursery school class joins a senior center club in their meeting room; once a month visits to a nursing home by primary grade children for a "party" planned to include specific activities in the recreation room; and shared holiday celebrations throughout the year for seniors and young children at a community day care center. Visitations must be carefully planned in each case so that no one is overtaxed by long trips or too much stimulation.

Ideally, the multi-generational groups should be equally balanced between youngsters and elders. But if this is not possible, then a group can function better if there are more children that if there are greater numbers of elderly.

The dance specialist or recreation coordinator will usually arrange and direct the sessions. It is helpful if individual group leaders and class teachers join in the planning and assist the participants during the activity. In order to provide appropriate content and smooth running sessions, it is best to prepare each group separately before meeting together. Structured games and dances may be even more successful if they are taught and practiced in advance.

The selection and progression of activities in each session will involve consideration of the abilities of the participants. Pre-school and primary age children are usually active with short attention spans. Independent elders may be quite vigorous, but most of the people in day centers and nursing homes tire easily or have some limitations which necessitate sitting activities and fairly moderate, simple movements. Therefore, resting and talking times, alternating singing and action games, or two part dances that allow for "taking turns" can be scheduled. The sessions may also be planned to include refreshments and time to perform for each other. Group members will appreciate the change of pace and the socializing opportunities.

A time period of forty minutes to an hour and a quarter is reasonable, depending upon the age and concentration abilities of the participants. Also, the activities should be varied and limited to three or four different ones at each meeting. Whenever arrangements are made to bring the age groups together, well laid plans facilitate creation of an atmosphere for joyful interaction.

Session Content

Sessions for combined age groups ideally include a variety of simple body motions to start and then progress to rhythmic games, creative movement, and group dancing. Participants can engage in stretching, shaking, tensing, thrusting, and swinging actions of their legs, arms and torsos for warm-up activities. These can be done in sideward, forward, backward, and circular directions. Variations may be devised to involve all group members, whether standing or sitting, ambulatory or chairbound. Double circles with the children in one and the elders in the other can accommodate varied energy and flexibility ranges. Pairing a youngster with an elderly person may inspire greater effort on the part of the older adult. Counting rhymes, such as "One, Two, Buckle My Shoes", "This Old Man", "One Fin-

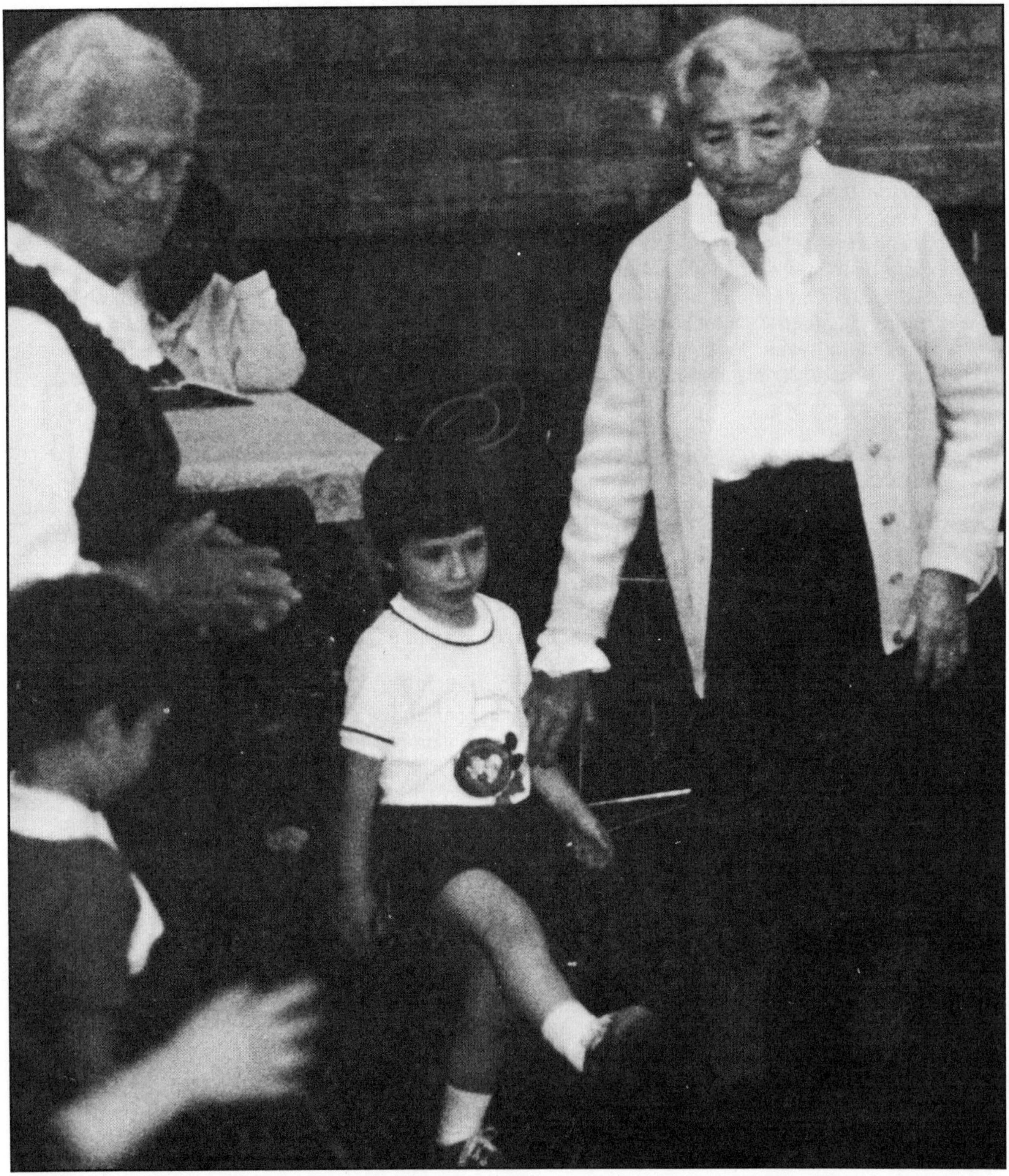

Creativity can be encouraged by using play party games such as "London Bridge" and folk dances like "Shoo Fly" and "Tarantella."

ger, One Thumb, Keep Moving" and finger plays like "The Eensie, Weensie Spider", "Little Peter Rabbit", "My Hat It Has Three Corners", "Wind, Wind, Wind Your Bobbin" and follow the leader activities such as "Simon Says", "Did You Ever See A Lassie", "Here We Go Round The Mulberry Bush", are all good ideas to use for developmental movement with intergenerational groups. (Nelson, 1973; Polk, 1972) The imagery and pantomime involved decrease the need for long, complicated explanations. Through these familiar rhythmic activities young and old participants may sing and help each other in a relaxed, playful manner while improving space concepts, coordination, flexibility and coordination skills.

Creativity can be encouraged by using play party games such as "London Bridge", "Here We Go Looby Loo", "Bridge of Avignon", "Alouette", "Row, Row, Row Your Boat" and folk dances like "Masquerade", "Cherkessia", "Shoo Fly", "Seven Jumps", "Mexican Waltz", "La Raspa", "Patch Tanz", "Tarantella", etc. (Barlin, 1974; Harris, et al, 1978; Lindner & Harpaz, 1982 & 1987). The elders and children can play different parts and share in ways that offer realistic challenges for each. More vigorous skipping, jumping, and running will be incorporated into the youngsters' dance responses, while the older adults will find expressive ways to join the dance pattern with clapping, stamping and rocking phrases. Physical contact between generations will often be a natural and enjoyable part of these movement responses.

Traditional folk dances typical of the ethnic backgrounds of the old and young group members may provide opportunities to pass on a cultural heritage and can emphasize the links between people from the past to the future. They may be performed with variations that use rhythm instruments, scarves, batons, and other props.

The children and older adults can also freely improvise to music, stories, poems, and other ideas. These dance activities usually result in cooperative decision making, expanded movement vocabulary, and joyful responses.

The quality of life for both generations can be enhanced through increased contact. As dance professionals, we can implement methods that can make these experiences richer and more fulfilling by providing social interaction and emotional sharing throughout the life span.

REFERENCE

Adelphi University. (1979). Love and learn. Videotape, Garden City, NY: Center on Aging.

Barlin, A. & Barlin, P. (1974). Dance-a-folk-song. Los Angeles, CA : Bowman.

Cohen, M.C., et al. (1981). The intergenerational caregiving program: A replication manual. San Francisco, CA: University of California School of Nursing.

Elvirita Lewis Foundation/Office of Child Development. (1978). Bridging generations: A handbook for intergenerational child care. CA: Department of Education.

Harris, J.A., Pittman, A.M., and Waller, M.S. (1978). Dance awhile. Minneapolis, MN: Burgess Publishing, fifth edition.

Kornhaber, A. and Woodward, K. (1981). Grandparents/grandchildren: The vital connection. Garden City, NY: Anchor/Doubleday.

Lindner, E.C., Harpaz, L. and Samberg, S. (1979). Therapeutic dance/movement: Expressive activities for older adults. New York, NY: Human Sciences.

Lindner, E. C. and Harpaz, L. (1987). Come dance again on your feet or in your seat. Baldwin, NY: Educational Activities.

Linder, E.C., and Harpaz, L. (1982). Special dancing on your feet or in your seat. Baldwin, NY: Educational Activities.

Nelson, E. (1973). Dancing games for children of all ages. NY: Sterling Publishing.

Nobel, N. Director, (1981). Close harmony. (Videotape), Washington, DC: Devillier-Donegan Enterprises, 9, NAT.

Parnell, K. (1980). "Young and old together: A review of the literature", Childhood Education, 56, pp. 184-188.

P.K. Yonge Laboratory School. (1976). From time to time: A record of young children's relationships with the aged. Gainsville, FL: University of Florida, Monograph #17, March.

Polk, Elizabeth. (1972). Orchestrated music for special children. NY: Hoctor Records.

Risso, S. and Mayo, C.R. (1979). "Games and kids could be the key", Journal of Health, Physical Education and Recreation, 50, (7), pp.34-35.

Seefeldt, C., Camp, S.B., Jantz, R.K. and Seerock, K. (1982). "How older people view children", Children Today, March-April.

Seefeldt, C., Camp, S.B., Jantz, R.K., and Seerock, K. (1979). Young and old together: A training manual for intergenerational programs. College Park, MD: University of Maryland.

VI. Resources

24

Selected Resources for Dance and the Older Adult

Josie Metal-Corbin

The following compilation of resources for dance and the older adult was gathered from a variety of sources. During the Spring of 1987, six hundred and fifty questionnaires were mailed or distributed to selected representatives of the following organizations:

1) The American Alliance for Health, Physical Education, Recreation and Dance (AAHPERD)
   a. National Dance Association (NDA)
   b. Council on Aging and Adult Development
   c. Research Consortium
   d. Participants from the NDA's Dance and the Older Adult Conferences, 1984 (New York University) and 1986 (Howard University)
   e. Presentors from AAHPERD Conventions, 1981-1987
   f. Authors who have published relevant articles in the Journal of Physical Education, Recreation and Dance since 1983.

2) The National Council on the Aging, Arts and Humanities Program

3) The National Association of Area Agencies on Aging

4) The Association for Gerontology in Higher Education (284 institutional representatives)

In addition, titles were selected from the Educational Resources Information Center (ERIC) and the Sport Information Resource Centre (SIRC) and a call for resources was published in the National Dance Association's publication Spotlight.

The questionnaire asked the respondent to: 1) identify classes, courses or workshops that focused on dance for the older adult; 2) identify teachers, leaders, and choreographers working with older adults, and 3) to recommend printed and non-print resources. The responses included information about modern, folk, tap, ballroom, square, belly, round, therapeutic, wheelchair, country western aerobic and aquatic dance.

Although this is not a comprehensive listing, every effort was made to conduct a thorough search. Any error or omission is unintentional. The author encourages suggestions and recommendations for future publications.

* This study would not have been possible without the support of the School of Health, Physical Education, and Recreation at the University of Nebraska at Omaha. The author is especially grateful to Sonia Green and Michael Stewart for their encouragement, to Nancy Glow, Kristi Nelson, Mary Beacom and Lou Meyers for their assistance in preparing this manuscript for press and to all the people who took the time to respond to the questionnaire.

BOOKS

Bechdahl, J. Dancing is a ball: A beginner's line dance manual. Keep Moving' of the USA, P.O. Box 512, Springfield, OH, 45501.

Beigel, L. (1984). Physical fitness and the older person: A guide to exercise for health care professionals. Rockville, MD: Aspen Systems Corp.

Chrisman, D. E. (1980). Body recall. Berea, KY: Berea College Press.

Coombs, J. (1981). Aerobic dance for the older adult. Canada: Recreation Development Division.

Corbin, D. E., & Metal-Corbin, J. (1983). Reach for it: A handbook of exercise and dance activities for older adults. Eddie Bowers Publishing, 2884 Hickory Hill, Dubuque, IA 52001.

deVries, H. (1974). Vigor regained. New Jersey: Prentice-Hall.

DePeters, Gordon, & Wertman. The magic of music. Saint Louis, MO: MMB Music, Inc., 10370 Page Industrial Boulevard, 68132.

Douglass, D. Accent on rhythm. Saint Louis, MO: MMB Music, Inc., 10370 Page Industrial Boulevard, 68132.

Garnet, E. D., (1982). Movement is life: A holistic approach to exercise for older adults. Princeton, NJ: Princeton Book Co.

Gomez, N., & Fortin, S. (1982). Danse et 1' apprentissage de comportements autonomes chey les personnes du troisieme age. Montreal: University de Montreal.

Gowitzke, B. (1981). Folk dance for the older adult. Canada: Recreation Development Division.

Kennedy, D. W., Austin, D. R., & Smith, R. W. (1987). Special recreation: Opportunities for persons with disabilities. Philadelphia: Saunders College Publishing.

Lang, D., & Stinson, W. Project towers resource guide: A wellness program for the elderly. Healthcomm, 2542 Westview Dr., Emporia, KS, 66801.

Lerman, L. (1984). Teaching dance to senior adults, Chicago, IL: Charles C. Thomas.

Levete, G. (1982). No handicap to dance: Creative improvisation for people with or without disabilities. London, England: Souvenir Press Ltd., U.S. Distributor, Brookline Books, 29 Ware Street, Cambridge, MA, 02138.

Lindner, E. C., Harpaz, L., & Samberg, S. (1979). Therapeutic dance/movement: Expressive activities for older adults. New York: Human Sciences Press.

Mettler, B. (1985). Dance as an element of life. Mettler Studios Inc., Tucson Creative Dance Center, 3131 North Cherry Ave., Tucson, AZ, 85719.

Nelson, E. (1973). Dancing games for children of all ages. New York: Sterling Publishers Co.

Price, W., & Lyon, L. (1987). A national directory of physical fitness programs for older adults, (2nd. ed.). North Country Community College Press, 20 Winona Ave., Saranac Lake, NY, 12983.

Sandel, S. L., & Kelleher, M. (1984). Dance/movement therapy. In L. Biegel (ed.), Physical fitness and the older person: A guide to exercise for health care professionals. (pp. 101-118). Rockville, MD: Aspen Systems Corp.

Schade, C., & Johnson, L. (1986). Prime time aerobics. 3089 C. Clairemont Dr., #130, San Diego, CA, 92117.

Schultz, S. (1980). Let's get moving: A fitness program developed for those over sixty. Mayville, ND: Mayville State College.

Stempfly, P. Keep movin'. Wonderhouse Press, P.O. Box 512, Springfield, OH, 45501.

Teaff, J. D. (1985). Leisure services with the elderly. St. Louis, IA: Times Mirror/Mosby College Publishing.

Thomson, C., & Warren, B. (Eds.). (1981). The thunder tree. Lancaster, England: LUDUS Dance Co.

Warren, B., & Nadeau, R. Using the creative arts in therapy: The power of the arts experience to expand human horizons. Cambridge, MA: Brookline Books.

SPECIAL PUBLICATIONS

Publications from The American Alliance For Health, Physical Education, Recreation and Dance, 1900 Association Drive, Reston, VA, 22091:

Beland, R. M. (1980). Service - Learning: Programs for the aging. A Guide to Practicum and Fieldwork Experiences in Health, Fitness, Dance and Leisure Services.

Cox, R. H. (1979). AAHPERD research consortium symposium papers: Health, fitness, recreation, and dance. A Research Report.

Dance for physically disabled persons: A manual for teaching ballroom, square, and folk dances to users of wheelchairs and crutches. (1976).

Fitt, S., & Riordan, A. (1980). Dance for the Handicapped: Focus on dance IX.

Fowler, C. B. (1977). Dance as education.

Hill, K. (1976). Dance for physically disabled persons.

Levitan, D. & Campanelli, L. Health, physical education, recreation, and dance for the older adult: A modular approach.

Mason, K. C. (1974). Dance therapy: Focus on dance VII.

Publications from The National Council on the Aging, Inc. (NCOA), 600 Maryland Ave., SW, West Wing 100, Washington, D.C., 20024:

Age, work and retirement: An annotated bibliography of publications and films, (1971-1981).

Balkema, J. (1986). The creative spirit: An annotated bibliography on the arts, humanities, and aging.

Cahill, P. (1981). Arts, the humanities and older Americans: A catalogue of program profiles.

Education: An arts/aging answer. (1980).

Hoffman, D. (1980). Pursuits of arts activities with older adults: An administrative and programmatic handbook.

Kaplan, M. (1983). Leisure, recreation, culture and aging: An annotated bibliography.

Kuykendall, T. J. (1980). Revitalize! A pilot program in arts/aging.

Layton, E. Through the looking glass. A visual statement (poster) on possibilities of creativity in old age.

Lewis-Kane, M., MacDicken, R., & McCutcheon, P. (1986). Older artist outreach: Project guidelines.

McCutcheon, P. B., & Bird, R. (1986). A manual for artists: How to find work in the field of aging.

McCutcheon, P. B., & Tecott, K. (1985). Developing older audiences: Guidelines for perform ing arts groups.

McCutcheon, P. B., & Wolf, C. S. (1984). Resource guide to people, places and programs in arts and aging.

Moody, R. (1982). Aging and cultural policy.

Service learning in aging: Implications for health, physical education, recreation and dance. (1982).

Ventura-Merkel, C. (1983). Cultural programs for and by older adults: A catalogue of program profiles.

Ventura-Merkel, C. (1983). Intergenerational programs: A catalogue of profiles.

SELECTED ARTICLES FROM PERIODICALS

Adams, D. (1983, May). Dance for older adults in a workshop setting. Journal of Physical Education, Recreation and Dance, 54, (5), 51.

Berryman-Miller, Sherrill, (1986). Benefits of Dance and the process of aging and Retirement for the older adult. Activities, Adaptation & Aging. Hawthorne Press.

Birren, J. E., et al. (1972). Research, demonstration, and training: Issues and methodology in social gerontology. The Gerontologist, 12, (2), 49-83.

Corbin, D. E., Kagan, D., & Metal-Corbin, J. (1987). A content analysis of an intergenerational unit on aging in a sixth grade classroom. Educational Gerontology: An Intergenerational Bimonthly Journal, 13, (5).

Dawson, A. and Baller, W. (1972). Relationship between creative activity and the health of elderly persons. Journal of Psychology., 82, 49-58.

Deborah, B. (1985). Effects of aerobic dance on physical work capacity, cardiovascular function and body composition of middle-age women. Research Quarterly for Exercise and Sport, 56, (3), 227-233.

Dennis, W. (1966). Creative productivity between ages of 20 to 80. The Journal of Gerontology, 21, 1-8.

Ensign, C. P. (1986). An interview with Liz Lerman. Journal of Physical Education, Recreation and Dance, 57, (1), 45.

Ensign, C. P. (1986, Jan.). An overview of dance. Journal of Physical Education, Recreation and Dance,
U57, (1), 45.

Fedirko, B., Hecox, B., Milliken, S., & Wilson, C. (1985). Dance as a p.t. modality: An experience in group treatment outside the hospital setting. Clinical Management in Physical Therapy, 5, (4), 44-47.

Goertzen, D., Serfass, R., Sopko, G., & Leon, A. (1984). The functional capacity and physical activity levels of women over 60 years of age. Journal of Sports Medicine and Physical Fitness, 24, (1), 30-36.

Hecox, B. (1983). Movement activities for older adults. Journal of Physical Education, Recreation and Dance, 54, (5), 47-48.

Hecox, B., Levine, E., & Scott, D. (1976). Dance in physical rehabilitation. Physical Therapy, 56, (8), 919-923.

Hecox, B., Levine, E., & Scott, D. (1976). Report on the use of dance in physical rehabilitation: Rehabilitation Literature, 36, (1), 11-16.

Helm, J. B. & Gill, K. L. (1974-75). An essential resource for the aging: Dance therapy. Dance Research Journal of C.O.R.D., 7, (1), 1-7.

Iannacone, G. & Skelly, J. (1985, May). Bridging the gap between senior citizens and young people. National Association of Secondary School Principals Bulletin, 69, (481), 99-101.

Jones, J. E. (1982). Gerontology and the arts. Educational Gerontology, 8, (2), 101-205.

Koss, R. (1986). Moving into the third age. AAHPERD serves a new clientele. Journal of Physical Education, Recreation and Dance, 57, (1), 30-31.

Lehman, H. (1958). The influence of longevity upon curves showing man's creative production rate at successive age levels. Journal of Gerontology, 13, 187-191.

Leviton, D. & Campanelli, L. C. (1984). Have we avoided the frail aged and dying older person in HPERD? Health Education, 15, (6), 43-47.

Lindner, E. C. (1982). Dance as a therapeutic intervention for the elderly. Journal of Educational Gerontology, 8, 167-174.

Lindner, E. C. & Harpaz, L. (1983). Shared movement programs: Children and older adults. Journal of Physical Education, Recreation and Dance, 54, (5), 49.

Lopez, R. (1983). Guidelines for using dance with older adults. Journal of Physical Education, Recreation and Dance, 54, (5), 44-45.

Meredith-Jones, B. (1961). Moving and living elderly people. Laban Art of Movement Guild Magazine, England, 27.

Metal-Corbin, J. (1983). Shared movement programs: College students and older adults. Journal of Physical Education, Recreation and Dance, 54, (5), 46,50.

Metal-Corbin, J. & Foltz, R. (1985). All my grandmothers could sing: An interdisciplinary and intergenerational choreographic work. Journal of Physical Education, Recreation and Dance, 55, (9), 52-55.

Missinne, L. & Lorenzen, L. Arts, the new wonder drug. Perspectives on Aging, 11, (3), 14-17.

Price, W. & Lyon, L. (1983). Fitness programs for the aged: A study of college and university involvement. Journal of Physical Education, Recreation and Dance, 54, (2), 42-44.

Pruett, D. M. (1983). Dance for older adults. Journal of Physical Education, Recreation and Dance, 54, (5), 43-51.

Schoenfeld, L. R. (1977, October). The psychomotor approach in the nursing home. Dance Magazine, 82-84.

Schoenfeld, L. R. (1975, March 3). A look at Americans in the year 2000. U.S. News and World Report.

Shea, M. M. (1986). Senior aerobics: Improving cardiovascular fitness. Journal of Physical Education, Recreation and Dance, 57, (1), 48-49.

PAPERS, MONOGRAPHS, PROCEEDINGS AND UNPUBLISHED MANUSCRIPTS

Anshel, M. H. (1985, April). Cognitive strategies to teach motor skills to elderly learners in nursing homes. Conference paper at the National Convention of the American Alliance of Health, Physical Education, Recreation and Dance.

Charles, R. F. (1981, January 23). A special programs adapted curriculum approach: Older adult education. Conference paper at the Conference of the Association of California Community College Administrators.

Corbin, D. E., Metal-Corbin, J., & Barker, G. (1987). Age doesn't matter: Weaving dance and aging into a fifth grade curriculum. (Document No. SP028013). Resources in Education, 22, 1. (ERIC No. ED 273623).

Irwin, K. (1972). Dance as a prevention of, therapy for, and recreation from the crisis of old age. A.D.T.A. Monograph No. 2, Columbia, Maryland: American Dance Therapy Association.

Koss, R. S. (1983, March). Aging and health - changing life-styles. Conference paper. Washington, D.C.: Administration on Aging (DHHS).

Lerman, L. (1982, October 14). Conference on expression of feelings through movement. Presented at Nebraska Psychiatric Institute, Omaha.

Lerman, L. (1981). Teaching modern dance to senior citizens: A manual. Unpublished thesis. George Washington University.

Palmer, M. K. (1985, November). Expressive therapists in long-term care settings. Conference paper at the National Conference of the American Association for Adult and Continuing Education.

Rabe, H. F. (1966, June). Training for new trends in clubs and centers for older persons. Proceedings of a seminar at Ithaca College. Albany, NY: New York State Education Dept.

Samberg, S. Therapeutic dance/movement. Unpublished manuscript. 5550 Fieldston Rd., Bronx, NY.

Sanwick, M. Rhythmic movement for the not so young. Unpublished manuscript. University of Nebraska-Lincoln.

Samuels, A. (1967). Dance for the aged: A.D.T.A. proceedings of the third annual conference. Columbia, Maryland: American Dance Therapy Association.

Strenger, L. A. & Smith, C. M. (1985, February). Healthy moves for older adults. Health, Physical Education, Recreation and Dance Monograph No. One (Report No., ISBN-0-89333-034-5). Washington, D.C.: ERIC Clearinghouse on Teacher Education.

Tinsley, Howard E. A. (1982). The psychological benefits of leisure activities for the elderly. Research report. Washington, D.C.: NRTA-AARP Andrus Foundation.

Research in Partial Fulfillment of the Requirements for the Master's Degree and the Doctoral Degree as compiled by Mary Alice Brennan in Research in Dance III (1982) sponsored by the National Dance Association.

MASTER'S DEGREE:

Fleishman, Ellen. (1977). The effect of movement therapy on the interactional behavior of geriatric patients with chronic organic brain syndrome: Three case studies. M.C.A.T., Hahnemann Medical College and Hospital.

Kelleher, M. (1978). Social interaction and affective expression in group movement therapy with the elderly. M.A., Wesleyen University.

Munns, Kathleen. (1978). The effects of a 12-week exercise and dance program on the range of joint motion of elderly subjects. M.S., University of Wisconsin at Madison.

Washington, Judy. (1978). Aquatic folkdance: An exercise unit for older adults. M.S., University of Wisconsin at Madison.

Weisbrot, Gwen. (1978). Senior citizens and dance. M.A., the American University.

Vapnek, Diane K. If you don't use it, you'll lose it: Creative movement with older adults. M.S., University of Georgia.

Zeidman, Barbara J. (1980). A study of movement therapy with geriatrics. M.A., Loyola Marymount University.

DOCTORAL DEGREE:

Boarman, Alice Marie. (1977). The effect of folk dancing upon reaction time and movement time of senior citizens. Ed.D., Oregon State University.

Holcomb, James Marion. (1977). The effects of dancing and relaxation sessions on stress levels of senior citizens. Ph.D., United States International University.

FILMS, VIDEOTAPES, SLIDES

A coming of age, (Film). (1976). SAGE Project. University of Minnesota, AV Library Service, 1313 Fifth St., S.E., Suite 108, Minneapolis, MN 55414.

Dance movement as therapy for older adults, (Film). American Dance Therapy Association, 2000 Century Plaza, Suite 108, Columbia, MD 21044.

Dance therapy: The power of movement, (Film). (1983). American Dance Therapy Association, 2000 Century Plaza, Suite 108, Columbia, MD 21044.

Dean, J. H. (Producer). (1980). The women of Hodson (Film). New York, NY: Filmmakers Library, Inc., 133 East 58 St., Suite 703A, 10022.

Don't take it easy. TV ONTARIO. University of Minnesota, AV Library Service, 1313 Fifth St., S.E., Suite 108, Minneapolis, MN 55414.

Griffith, B. R., & Martin, P. Sodanceabit, (Videotape, Manual). 1401 Anaheim Place, Long Beach, CA 90804.

Health, fitness and leisure for a quality life. (20 min. film). American Alliance for Health, Physical Education, Recreation and Dance, NEA Sound Studios, 1900 Association Drive, Reston, VA 22091.

Leviton, D. (Producer), and Callahan, G. (Director). Smiles: The adults' health and developmental program. (Film). College Park, MD: Adult Health and Development Program, PEHR Building, University of Maryland, 20740.

Metal-Corbin, J. (Project Director), Bottum, D. (Director/Producer), & Corbin, D. E. (Writer/Narrator). (1985). Age doesn't matter: Weaving dance and aging into a fifth grade curriculum. (Videotape). University Television, University of Nebraska at Omaha, Omaha, NE 68182.

Metal-Corbin, J. (Director/Choreographer), Langdon, J. (Producer/Director), & Greenblatt, D. (Composer). (1986). Out of the shadow, into the light. (Videotape). A concert dance for older women. University Television, University of Nebraska at Omaha, Omaha, NE 68182.

Metal-Corbin, J. (Project Director), Scollon, W. (Director/Producer). (1983). Old friends: An intergenerational approach to dance. (Videotape). University Television, University of Nebraska at Omaha, Omaha, NE 68182.

Metal-Corbin, J. (Director/Choreographer), Scollon, W. (Producer/Director), & Foltz, R. (Composer). (1985). All my grandmothers could sing. (Videotape). A concert dance for older women. University Television, University of Nebraska at Omaha, Omaha, NE 68182.

Mettler, B. (1970). The art of body movement. (Film). Tucson, AZ: Mettler Studios, Inc., 3131 North Cherry Ave., Tucson, AZ, 85719.

Riordan, A. A very special dance. (VHS cassette or film). AAHPERD Publications, 1900 Association Drive, Reston, VA 22091.

ROM Dance. (Videotape, Manual). Central Chapter of the Arthritis Foundation, 2501 North Star Road, Columbus, OH 43221.

Yahnke, R. The great circle of life: A guide to films on aging. (1987). The General College, 106 Nicholson Hall, 216 Pillsburg Dr., S.E., Minneapolis, MN, 55455. To be published by Rynd Publications in 1987.

RECORDS, AUDIOCASSETTES, MANUALS

Addison, C. Fifty positive vigor exercises for senior citizens. AAHPERD, American Alliance Publications, 1900 Association Drive, Reston, VA 22091.

Alberts, C. And the beat goes on. (Record Album LP 5020). Educational Activities, Box 392, Freeport, NY 11520.

Bell, R. D. et al. Reaching for the sun. Health Association, 440 Cambie Street, Vancouver, B.C. V6B 2N6, Canada.

Benison, B. The magic of movement. (Activities for those with limited movement). Melody House Publications Co., 819 N.W. 92nd St., Oklahoma City, OK, 73114.

Garnet, E. D. (1982). Chair exercise manual: An audio assisted program. Princeton Book Co., Princeton, NJ.

Gibbs, N. Wheels, reels, and squares. (Record Album). American Health Care Association, 1200 15th Street N.W., Washington, D.C. 20005.

Goldsmith, C. Relaxation: The key to life. (Record Album, LP 9080). Educational Activities, Box 392, Freeport, NY 11520.

Lindner, E. C. & Harpaz, L. (1987). Come dance again on your feet or in your seat. (Record, cassette, manual). P.O. Box 993, Woodside, NY 11377.

Lindner, E. C., & Harpaz, L. Special music for special people. (Record, cassette, manual). P.O. Box 993, Woodside, NY 11377.

Lindner, E. C., & Harpaz, L. Special dancing - On your feet or in your seat. (Record, cassette, manual). P.O. Box 993, Woodside, NY 11377.

MacCallum, M. Choreographed aerobic fitness for active older Canadians. (Cassette and Instructional Manual). 905 Standard Life Center, 10405 Jasper Ave., Edmonton, Alberta, Canada, T5J 3N4.

Memory Lane. Melody House Publication Co., 819 N.W. 92 St., Oklahoma City, OK 73114.

Sobul, A. L. Modified exercises for senior adults. MESA, 3555 Tolland Road, Shaker Heights, OH 44120.

PROGRAM AND RESOURCE PEOPLE

Ken Aldrich
531 Flamingo
Springfield, OR 97477

Janell Andrews
1005 North Sunset Drive
Olathe, KS 66061

June Andrus
Andrus Fitness, Inc.
Water Exercise Fitness
351 Scott Drive
Silver Spring, MD 20904

Pearl Atkinson
4621 SW Patton Rd.
Portland, OR 97221

Marcia Bagby
Country Western
Gainesville Parks and Recreation
850 Green Street
Gainesville, GA 30501

Mary Pat Balkus
Radford University
Box 5734
Radford, VA 24141

D. L. Timble Barber
Modern Dance & Ballet
Pasadena City College
1570 E. Colorado Blvd.
Pasadena, CA 91106

Ann Barton
Modern Dance
Sweden Senior Center
133 State St.
Brockport, NY 14420

Rayma K. Beal
Dance Activities for the Older Adult
University of Kentucky
Department of Health, Physical Education and Recreation
Seaton Building
Lexington, KY 40506

Jean Beckdahl's
Deepa Dancin'
Keep Movin' of the U.S.A.
P.O. Box 512
Springfield, OH 45501

Betty Sue Benison
Country Western & Folk Dance
Texas Christian University
P.O. Box 32901
Ft. Worth, TX 76129

Sherrill Berryman-Miller
Kinetic Movement and Social Dance
Howard University
Dance Division, Department of Physical Education and Recreation
4903 New Hampshire Ave., N.W.
Washington, D.C. 20011

Dee Ann Birkel
Ball State University
Retirees' Wellness Program
Ball Gym
Muncie, IN 47306

Ann Brekke
Social and Square Dance
Senior Citizen Center
Mayville, MO 64468

Cecelia Brown
Ballroom Dance
University of Wisconsin-Oshkosh
Kolf Sports Center
Oshkosh, WI 54901

Sandra Bruce
Older Americans' Center
Dances & Dance Instruction
349 S. Walnut
Bloomington, IN 47401

Victoria Buchler
Dancecise and Modern Dance
United Federation Of Teachers
Retired Teachers' Chapter
260 Park Avenue South
New York, NY

Jane Buechtel
Keep Dancin'
Elderly United
1 Fountain Square
Springfield, OH 45501

Virginia Carver
Movement For Older Adults
Georgia Center For Continuing Education
University of Georgia
Athens, GA 30602

Gail Chew
Tap, Aerobic, and Square Dance
University of Missouri - St. Louis
Active Adult Program
8001 Natural Bridge Rd.
St. Louis, MO 63121

David E. Corbin
Reach For It (exercises, dance, health)
University of Nebraska at Omaha
School of HPER
Omaha, NE 68182

Letty Delaney
King James Care Center
Dance For Wheel-Chair Bound Women
133 Hobart Rd.
Summit, Nj 07901

Carol Downs
Movement For Older Adults
Georgia Center For Continuing Education
University of Georgia
Athens, GA 30602

Randi Dressel
Social Dancing With Alzheimer's Disease Patients
Odd Fellows & Rebekah Nursing Home
104 Old Niagra Road
Lockport, NY 14094

Roland Dupree
School Of Dance
8115 W. Third Street
Los Angeles, CA 90048

Beht Eastuly
Chance To Dance
863 Pine Hill Rd.
Westport, MA 02790

Cynthia Ensign
Aerobic Dance
University of Northern Iowa
East Gym 107- School of HPER
Cedar Falls, IA 50614

Denise M. Frazee
Aeorbic Dance Program
Human Development Center
Delta College
University Center, MI 48710

Pauline Fisher
Particinformance
Audience Participation In Exercise And Dance
1884 Columbia Rd. NW #105
Washington, DC 20009

Flo Garrett
Folk Dance And Body Movement
University of Delaware
2800 Pennsylvania Ave.
Wilmington, DE 19806

James German
Ballroom Dancing
5623 Ravenel Lane
Springfield, MA 22151

Sheila Gilstein
Intro to Dance/Movement Therapy
Department of Dance
Brookdale Community College
Newman Springs Rd.
Lincroft, NJ 07738

Robin Graham
Relaxation, Improvisation, Folk Dance
68 W. 10 St. Apt. 30
New York, NY 10011

The Grande Olde Players Company
A Performing Dramatic Troupe Including
A Dance Line, "The Grande Dancers"
4909 Dodge St.
Omaha, NE 68132

Betty Rose Griffith
Sodanceabit
Social Dance Aerobics
1401 Anaheim Place
Long Beach, CA 90804

Susan Grotts
Tap Dance
San Carlos Senior Center
601 Chestnut
San Carlos, CA 94070

Janice Baker Haines
Orchesis II Dance Club, Working With Older Adults
240 PEB
Iowa State University
Ames, IA 50011

Leah Harpaz
Elders Share The Arts Program
Dance/Movement/Exercise: Classes For Parkinson's Disease Patients In Long Island
Fall Workshop And Classes at 92nd Street, YMYWHA
Dance & Physical Activities For Older Adults: Course At Adelphi University
C.U.E. Program Of Queens College
P.O. Box 993
Woodside, NY 11377

Bernadette Hecox
Physical Therapy Program - Dance With Arthritis And Parkinson's Disease Patients
Columbia University
630 W. 168 St.
New York, NY 10032

Carol Horwitz
Chataqua Program At Cornell College And Elderhostel Program
Mt. Vernon, IA
711 2nd Avenue
Iowa City, IA 52240

Marilyn Huber
Athrocize-Aerobic Dance
Michiana Fitness Services
P.O. Box 2314
South Bend, IN 46614

Wallace Hutchinson
Aerobic Dance
Iowa State University
240 PEB
Ames, IA 50011

Gwen Hyatt
Desert Southwest Fitness, Inc.
Moderate Motion Workshop, Aerobic Dance
1054 Lamplighter Drive
Logan, UT 84321

Bernard "Skeeter" Johnson
GeroFitness
University of Kentucky Center On Aging
120 Seaton Bldg.
University of Kentucky
Lexington, KY 40506

Eileen Jones
Laban Based Movement With Older Adults
225 E. 5 Street
New York, NY 10003

Billie Kirpich
Movement For Health
c/o Muse Isle Senior Center
2501 M.W. 16 St. Rd.
Miami, FL 33125

Laura Knox
Southern Danceworks
2717 7th Ave. South
Birmingham, AL 35233

Liz Lerman
Dance Exchange
Dancers Of The Third Age
P.O. Box 40909
Washington, DC 20016

Dan Leviton
Adult Health And Development Program
University of Maryland
PERH Bldg., Suite 2387
College Park, MD 20742

Pam Lewis
Energy Hour, Exercise By The Sea
88 Pkwy. S. Apt. A
New London, CT 06320

Peggy Lewis
Clogging, Square Dance, Ballroom, Folk
Good Life Resort
Mesa, AZ 85206

Karen Lieterman
Tai Chi
Las Cruces Family YMCA
P.O. Box 16453
Las Cruces, NM 88004

Erna Caplow Lindner
Dance/Movement/Exercise Classes For Parkinson's Disease Patients In Long Island
Fall Workshop at 92nd Street, YMYWHA
Courses Taught At Adelphi University And Nassau Community College
C.U.E. Program Of Queens College
Elders Share The Arts Program
P.O. Box 993
Woodside, NY 11377

Long Beach Parks & Recreation
Round, Square, Swing, Tap, Social Classes
P.O. Box 15827
Long Beach, CA 90815

Maggie Loridas
Round, Tap, Belly, Square, and Group Dances
City of Farmington Hills - Sr. Adult Services
31555 Eleven Mile Rd.
Farmington Hills, MI 48018

Margaret Mains
1308 Grand Ave.
Laramie, WY 82070

Alice Markwood
Movement Therapy - YWCA
2361 Westchester Blvd.
Springfield, IL 62704

Marjory Marsh
Aerobic Dance
1632 Moon St., N.E.
Albuquerque, NM 87112

Marjory Marsh
Lite-Line Exercise For Older Adults, Methods Of Teaching Aerobic Dance
HPER Department
University of New Mexico
Albuquerque, NM 87131

Carol McGinn
Ballroom Dance Club
Iowas State University
240 PEB
Ames, IA 50011

Billie McKenzie
Sit And Be Fit & Surviving Aerobics
2390 Harrison Dr.
Dunedin, FL 33528

Rose Medina
Chairxercise, Over Easy
Metamorphosis
1309 Foster
Las Cruces, NM 88001

Josie Metal-Corbin
Reach For It (exercise, dance)
University of Nebraska At Omaha
School of HPER
Omaha, NE 68182

Muriel Miller
Folk Dance
Senior Centers In Mesa, Scottsdale
1325 Leisure World
Mesa, AZ 85206

Fred & Ruth Minster
Clogging and Square Dance
Delta College
University Center, MI 48710

Alice Newbold
Swing Into Shape
1815 Coventry Dr.
Champaign, IL 61821

Sue Newell
Wheel Chair/Adapted Dancing
717 Harrison St.
Council Bluffs, IA 51501

Angela Nicolosi
Dance/Movement Exercise Program With National Arthritis Foundation
161 W. Hubbard Ave. #205
Columbus, OH 43215

Ruth Nobel
Dance Classes
589 S.O.M. Center Rd. (Rt. 91)
Solon, OH 44139

Paul Oertel
Problems In Movement/Dance
Naropa Institution
2130 Arapahoe
Boulder, CO 80302

Nancy Osgood
Researcher, Program Planning Specialist In Dance As Therapy With Older Adults
Gerontology Department
MCV Station 28
Richmond, VA 23298-001

Cas Overton
Tai Chi
Virginia Commonwealth University
Department of Dance
1315 Floyd Ave.
Richmond, VA 23228

Ralph Piper
Resource Person For Dance Classes In Leisure World
3123-D Via Serena North
Laguna Hills, CA 92653

Margaret J. Pope
Dance For A Special Population
Jacksonville State University
Jacksonville, AL 36265

John Ramsay
Folk, English Country, Period Dance
Berea College
Recreation Extension
Berea, KY 40404

Julee Richardson
Tap Dance, Jazz Dance
Quest
Chabot College Hayward Campus
25555 Hesperian Blvd.
Hayward, CA 94545

Roberta Richardson
Alive! Prime Timers
Bethesda/Chevy Chase YMCA
Old Georgetown Rd.
Bethesda, MD 20814

Vicki Roitman
The Silver Streak Dancers
Jewish Community Center Of Greater Kansas City
6201 Indian Creek
Overland Park, KS 66207

Gail Rollow
Over 40 Aerobic Exercise And Dance
Congress Hall-Life Long Learning Center
8150 N. Congress
Kansas City, MO 64152

Marilyn Roman
Movement of Fitness
Center for Aging
University of Alabama in Birmingham
933 S. 19 St.
Birmingham, AL 32505

Karen Ross
Group Dances
Madonna College
36600 Schoolcraft
Livonia, MI 48150

Patricia Rowe
New York University
Department of Dance, Dance Education
35 W. 4th Street, 675
New York, NY 10003

Lucy A. Sack
Introduction to Creative Dance
Slippery Rock University
110 Morrow Fieldhouse
Slippery Rock, PA 16057

Cindy Scarborough
Movement Classes For Alzheimer's Patients And Sight-Impaired Okder Adults
New York University
Dance Education Department
35 W. 4 St.
New York, NY 10003

Charlene J. Schade
Exhibition Dance, Prime Time Aerobics
5205 Mount Alifan Drive
San Diego, CA 92111

Susan Schultz
Geriokinesiatrics
North Dakota State University, Mayville
Mayville, ND 58257

Tish Searcy
Ballroom Dance
Gainesville Junior College
P.O. Box 1358
Gainesville, GA 30503

Elaine Shafrin
Center On Arts And Aging
Research Assistant
600 Maryland Ave., SW
West Wing 100
Washington, DC 20024

Marianne M. Shea
Biogerontology Laboratory
504 N. Walnut Street
University of Wisconsin-Madison
Madison, WI 53706

Allen Sher
62 Meadow Brook Rd.
Rutland, VT 05701

Andria Sherman
Dance For The Older Adult
New York University
Dance Education Department
35 W. 4th St.
New York, NY 10003

Everett L. Smith
The Biogerontology Laboratory
University of Wisconsin - Madison
504 N. Walnut Street
Madison, WI 53705

Maargaret E. Smith
Researcher, Program Planning Specialist On
Dance As Therapy With Older Adults
8701 Beacontree Lane, Apt. 7
Richmond, VA 23229

Arlynne Stark
Goucher College
Dept. Of Dance/Movement Therapy
Goucher College
Towson, MD 21204

Michael Steele
Ballroom Dancing
8150 N. Congress
Kansas City, MO 64152

Rose Strasser & Datus Herzog
Tap, Folk, Ballroom, Aerobics and Square Dance
Tower Point Resort
Mesa, AZ 85206

Marietta Suhart
The Georgia Center For Continuing Education
The University of Georgia
Athens, GA 30602

Jackie Tally
Eldercise-Lloyd Noldan Hospital And
Southern Danceworks
2717 7th Ave. South
Birmingham, AL 35233

Andrea Tecza
Beginning Modern Dance, "Senior Guests"
Dance Unit
School of PER & D
Kent State University
Kent, OH 44242

Marcie Telander
Drama & Creative Movement
2005 N. Mohawk
Chicago, IL 60614

Delfa Malvagni Vasnaugh
1884 Columbia Rd. NW
Washington, DC 20009

Caroline Walter
Ballroom & Aerobic
Towson State University
Towson, MD 21204

Eleanor B. Wapner
GRN 127 Movement Therapy Course
Malloy College
1000 Hempstead Ave.
Rockville Centre, NY 11570

Michele Whitlatch
Desert Southwest Fitness, Inc.
Moderate Motion Workshop, Aerobic Dance
5330 E. Golden Ranch
Tucson, AZ 85704

Teresa Young
Young At Heart Lifetime Fitness
107 N. Main
Lansing, KS 66043

Phyl Yates
Lincoln Center For Seniors
1435 "0" St.
Lincoln, NE 68508

Ben Zalas
Dempsey Hall
800 Algoma Bldg.
Oshkosh, WI 54901

CHOREOGRAPHERS

June M. Andrus
Andrus Fitness Inc.
351 Scott Drive
Silver Spring, MD 20904

Rachelle Ava & Robert Teri
Joy Of Motion Dance Center, Inc.
1643 Conneticut Ave., N.W.
Washington, DC 20009

Ann Barton
Modern Dance
Sweden Senior Center
133 State St.
Brockport, NY 14420

Teresa Benzwie
Free Lance Movement Consultant
1244 Forge Rd.
Cherry Hill, NJ 08034

Victoria Buchler
155 W. 68 St.
New York, NY 10023

Sally Charnon
Elders Share the Arts
425 E. 25 #825
New York, NY 10010

Gail Chew
University of Missouri at St. Louis
Physical Education Department
8001 Natural Bridge Rd.
St. Louis, MO 13121

Lynn Coles
Quest - Expanding Education For Elders (50 and up)
Chabot College - Hayward Campus
25555 Hesperian Blvd.
Hayward, CA 94545

Sage Cowles
247 10th Ave. South
Minneapolis, MN 55415

Letty Delaney
King James Care Center
133 Hobart Rd.
Summitt, NJ 07901

Beth Eastuly
Chance To Dance
863 Pine Hill Rd.
Westport, MA 02790

Denise M. Frazee
Human Development Center
Devising An Aerobic Dance Program For Older Adults
Delta College
University Center, MI 48710

Mr. & Mrs. James German
Forward Step, Inc.
5623 Ravonel Lance
Springfield, MA 22151

Anita Glick
Private Work With Older Adults
2467 St. 10
Bldg. 21 Apt 8-B
Morris Plains, NJ 07950

Robin Graham
68 W. 10 St. #30
New York, NY 10011

Janice Baker Haines
Lifemoves
240 PEB
Iowa State University
Ames, IA 50011

Leah Harpaz
Elders Share The Arts
425 E. 25 #825
New York, NY 10010

Jacelyn Helm
Princeton Senior Resource Center
Spruce Circle
Princeton, NY 08540

Carol Horwitz
Chataqua Program
Cornell College
Mt. Vernon, IA 52314

Jefferson James
Contemporary Dance Theatre
2728 Vine
Cincinnati, OH 45219

Susan Perlstein
Elder Share The Arts
424 E. 25 #825
New York, NY 10010

Marilyn Richardson
Department of HPER
South Dakota State University
Brookings, SD 57006

Peggy Ryan
Peggy Ryan & The TNT Dancers
3427 S. Eastern Pkwy.
Las Vegas, NV 89109

Cindy Scarborough
Prime Time: Seniors In Motion Dance Company
Janus Dance Projects, Inc.
15 S. William Street
New York, NY 10004

Susan Schultz
State University of North Dakota at Mayville
Mayville, ND 58257

Marion Scott
969 Hilgard Ave.
Penthouse #4
Los Angeles, CA 90024

Michael Steele
8150 N. Congress
Kansas City, MO 64152

Jackie Tally & Laura Knox
Southern Danceworks
2717 7th Ave., South
Birmingham, AL 35233

Delfa Malvagni Vasnaugh
1884 Columbia Rd. NW
Washington, DC 20009

Caroline Walter
Towson State University
Towson, MD 21204

Billie Kirpich
Performing Group
111 N.W. First Street
Miami, FL 33128-1985

Liz Lerman
Dance Exchange, Dancers Of The Third Age
P.O. Box 40909
Washington, DC 20016

Pam Lewis
88 Parkway S. Apt. A
New London, CT 06320

Erna Caplow Lindner
Elders Share The ARts
425 E. 25th St. #825
New York, NY 10010

Maggie Loridas
31555 Eleven Mile Rd.
Farmington Hills, MI 48018

Alice Markwood
Y-Not Dancers, YWCA
421 E. Jackson St.
Springfield, IL 62701

Margie Marsh
1632 Moon St. N.E.
Alburquerque, NM 87112

Billie McKenzie
2390 Harrison Dr.
Dunedin, Fl 33528

Josie Metal-Corbin
University of Nebraska at Omaha
School of HPER
Omaha, NE 68182

Louise Mattlage
c/o Calyx Books
P.O. Box B
Corvallis, OR 97339

Tova Orbeck
N. 3 Lighthouse Rd.
Big Bay, MI 49808

PERIODICALS

Activities, Adaptation & Aging
Haworth Press, Inc.
28 E. 22nd St.
New York, NY 10010

Aging
U.S. Government Printing Office
Washington, DC 20402

Aging Alert
CD Publications
100 Summit Bldg.
8555 16th St., Suite 100
Silver Spring, MD 20910

Aging and Work
National Council on the Aging, Inc.
600 Maryland Ave., S.W., West Wing 100
Washington, DC 20024

Aged Care and Services Review
The Haworth Press, Inc
28 E. 22nd St.
New York, NY 10010

Aging International
International Federation on Aging
1909 K. St., N.W.
Washington, DC 20049

Aging and Society
Cambridge University Press
32 E. 57th St.
New York, NY 10022

American Geriatrics Society Journal
W.B. Saunders Co.
West Washington Square
Philadelphia, PA 19105

Clinical Gerontologist
The Haworth Press, Inc.
28 E. 22nd St.
New York, NY 10010

Concern in Care of the Aging
American Association of Homes for the Aging
1050 17th St., N.W., Suite 770
Washington, DC 20036

Generations
Western Gerontological Society
833 Market St., Suite 516
San Francisco, CA 94103

Geriatrics
Harcourt Brace Jovanovich, Inc.
One E. First St.
Duluth, MN 55802

Geriatric Nursing
American Journal of Nursing
555 W. 57th St.
New York, NY 10019

Gerontologist
Gerontological Society of America
1411 K St., N.W., Suite 300
Washington, DC 20005

Gerontology and Geriatrics Education
University of Texas Press
P.O. Box 7819
Austin, TX 78712

Gray Panthers Network
Gray Panthers
3700 Chestnut St.
Philadelphia, PA 19104

International Journal of Aging & Human Development
Baywood Publishing Co., Inc.
120 Mrina St., Box D
Farmingdale, NY 11735

International Social Security Review
International Social Security Association
Case Postale 1, CH-1211
Geneva 22, Switzerland

Journal of the American Geriatrics Society
W.B. Saunders Co.
W. Washington Square
Philadelphia, PA 19105

Journal of Applied Gerontology
University of South Florida
P.O. Box 3183
Tampa, FL 33620

Journal of Gerontological Nursing
C.V. Slack, Inc.
6900 Grove Rd.
Thorofare, NJ 08086

Journal of Gerontological Social Work
The Haworth Press, Inc.
28 E. 22nd St.
New York, NY 10010

Journal of Long-Term Care Administration
The American College of Nursing Home Administrators
4650 East-West Highway
P.O. Box 5890
Washington, DC 20014

Journal of Minority Aging
National Council on Black Aging, Inc.
Box 8813
Durham, NC 27707

Journal of Nutrition for the Elderly
The Haworth Press, Inc.
28 E. 22nd St.
New York, NY 10010

Leisure Information Quarterly
New York University
635 East Building
Washington Square
New York, NY 10003

Lifelong Learning
Adult Education Association of the U.S.A.
1201 16th St., N.W., Suite 301
Washington, DC 20036

Modern Maturity
American Association of Retired Persons
1901 K St., N.W.
Washington, DC 20026

Modern Nursing Homes
American Nursing Home Association
1200 15th St., N.W.
Washington, Dc 20005

S.A.G.E.
Project News
National Association for Humanistic Gerontology
Claremont Office Part
41 Tunnel Rd.
Berkeley, CA 94705

Nursing Homes
American Nursing Home Association
1200 15th St., N.W.
Washington, DC 20005

Omegaa
Journal of Death and Dying
Baywood Publishing Co., Inc.
42 Central Dr.
Farmingdale, NY 11735

Physical and Occupational Therapy in Geriatrics
The Haworth Press, Inc.
28 E. 22nd St.
New York, NY 10010

Research on Aging
Sage Publications Inc.
275 S.
Beverly Hills, CA 90212

Retirement Life
National Association of Retired Federal Employees
1533 New Hampshire Ave., N.W.
Washington, DC 20036

Social Security Bulletin
U.S. Government Printing Office
Washington, DC 20402

Social Work in Health Care
The Haworth Press, Inc.
28 E. 22nd St.
New York, NY 10010

Journal of Geriatric Psychiatry
International Universities Press, Inc.
315 Fifth Avenue
New York, NY 10016

AGENCIES AND ORGANIZATIONS

Administration on Aging
Department of Health and Human Services
Washington, DC 20201

American Academy of Geriatric Dentistry
2 N. Riverside Plaza
Chicago, IL 60603

American Alliance for Health, Physical Education, Recreation and Dance
Council on Aging and Adult Development
1900 Association Drive
Reston, VA 22091

American Association for Geriatric Psychiatry
230 N. Michigan Ave., Suite 2400
Chicago, IL 60601

American Association of Homes of the Aging
1050 17th St., N.W., Suite 770
Washington, DC 20036

American Association of Retired Persons
1909 K St., N.W.
Washington, DC 20049

American College of Nursing Home Administrators
4650 East-West Highway
Washington, DC 20014

American Dance Therapy Association, Inc.
2000 Century Plaza, Suite 230
Columbia, MD 21044

American Geriatrics Society
10 Columbus Circle
New York, NY 10019

American Public Health Association
Section on Gerontological Health
1015 18 St., N.W.
Washington, DC 20036

American Psychiatric Association
Council on Aging
1700 18 St., N.W.
Washington, DC 20009

American Psychological Association
Division of Adult Development and Aging
1200 17 St. , N.W.
Washington, DC 20036

American Nurses Association, Inc.
Council of Nursing Home Nurses
Division on Gerontological Nursing Practice
2420 Pershing Rd.
Kansas City, MO 64108

American Nursing Home Association
1200 15th St., N.W.
Washington, DC 20005

American Society on Aging
(formerly Western Gerontological Society)
833 Market St., Suite 516
San Fancisco, CA 94103

Arts for Elders
Theater Group
5450 S.W. Erickson Ave.
Beaverton, OR 97005

Arts and Humanities Program
National Council on the Aging
600 Maryland Ave., S.W., #200
Washington, DC 20024

Asian and Pacific Coalition on Aging
1851 S.W. Moreland Ave.
Los Angeles, CA 90006

Association for Humanistic Gerontology
1711 Solano Ave.
Berkeley, CA 94707

Association Canadienne de Gerotologie
Canadian Association on Gerontology
722 16th Ave., N.E.
Calgary, Alberta T2E 6V7

Association for Gerontology in Higher Education
600 Maryland Ave., S.W.
West Wing 204
Washington, DC 20024

Associacion National Por Personas Mayores
National Association for Spanish Speaking Elderly
3875 Wilshire Blvd., Suite 1401
Los Angeles, CA 90010

Center for the Study of Aging
706 Madison Ave.
Albany, NY 12208

ESTA
Elders Share The Arts, Inc.
425 E. 25 Street, Rm. 825
New York, NY 10010

Elderhostel
100 Boylston St.
Suite 200
Boston, MA 02116

Ethel Percy Andrus Gerontology Center
University of California
Los Angeles, CA 90007

Gray Panthers
3635 Chestnut St.
Philadelphia, PA 19104

International Federation on Aging
1909 K St., N.W.
Washington, DC 20006

International Senior Citizens' Association, Inc.
11753 Wilshire Blvd.
Los Angeles, CA 90025

Leadership Council of Aging Organizations
c/o Jack Ossofsky
National Council on Aging
600 Maryland Ave.
West Wing 100
Washington, DC 20024

National Association of Area Agencies on Aging
600 Maryland Ave., Suite 208
Washington, DC 20024

National Association for Human Development
1750 Pennsylvania Ave., N.W.
Washington, DC 20066

National Association of Mature People
918 16th St., N.W.
Washington, DC 20006

National Association of Nutrition and Aging Services
1601 Second Ave., Suite 800
Seattle, WA 98101

National Association of Retired Federal Employees
1533 New Hampshire Ave., N.W.
Washington, DC 20036

National Center on Rural Aging
c/o National Council on the Aging
600 Maryland Ave., S.W,
West Wing 100
Washington, DC 20024

National Citizens' Coalition for Nursing Home Reform
1424 16th St., N.W., Suite 204
Washington, DC 20036

National Committee on Careers for Older Americans
1414 22nd St., N.W., Room 602
Washington, DC 20037

National Council on the Aging, Inc.
600 Maryland Ave., S.W.
Washington, DC 20024

National Geriatric Society
212 W. Wisconsin Ave.
Milwaukee, WI 53203

National Institute on Adult Daycare
600 Maryland Ave., S.W.
West Wing 100
Washington, DC 20024

National Institute of Senior Citizens
c/o National Council on the Aging
600 Maryland Ave., S.W.
West Wing 100
Washington, DC 20024

National Interfaith Coalition on Aging
P.O. Box 1904
Athens, GA 30602

National Voluntary Organization for Independent
Living for the Aging
600 Maryland Ave., S.W.
West Wing 100
Washington, DC 20024

Older Women's League
1325 6 St., N.W.
Lower Level B
Washington, DC 20005

Retired Officers Association
1625 I St., N.W.
Washington, DC 20006

Retired Professional Action Group
200 P St., N.W., Suite 711
Washington, DC 20001

Senior PAC
1302 18th St., N.W.
Washington, DC 20036

Southern Gerontological Society
Gerontology Center
Georgia State University
Atlanta, GA 30303

Urban Elderly Coalition
1828 St., N.W.
Washington, DE 20036

25

1984 and 1986 Dance Conferences

The Multifaceted Roles Of Dance For The Older Adult

Sherrill Berryman-Miller

The first Eastern Division Conference to explore the role of dance in serving the burgeoning population of older adults was held at New York University, December 8, 1984. The conference was co-sponsored by the Department of Dance and Dance Education, New York University and the National Dance Association of AAPHERD. It was coordinated by Professor Judith G. Schwartz of New York University and Dr. Margie Hanson, Executive Director of the National Dance Association.

A second conference on current research and practical application of physical activities for older adults was coordinated by Dr. Sherrill Berryman-Miller and held on October 18, 1986, at Howard University. The program was co-sponsored by Howard University Wide Cultural Committee and the National Dance Association.

Each conference included panelists, workshop leaders and participants involved in the field of addressing and servicing the physical, psychological, and social needs in the aging process of the older adult.

The key ideas that came out of the conferences were:

- Movement can make a significant and important contribution both to the older adult and society as a whole.
- The older adult is the fastest growing population segment in the United States.

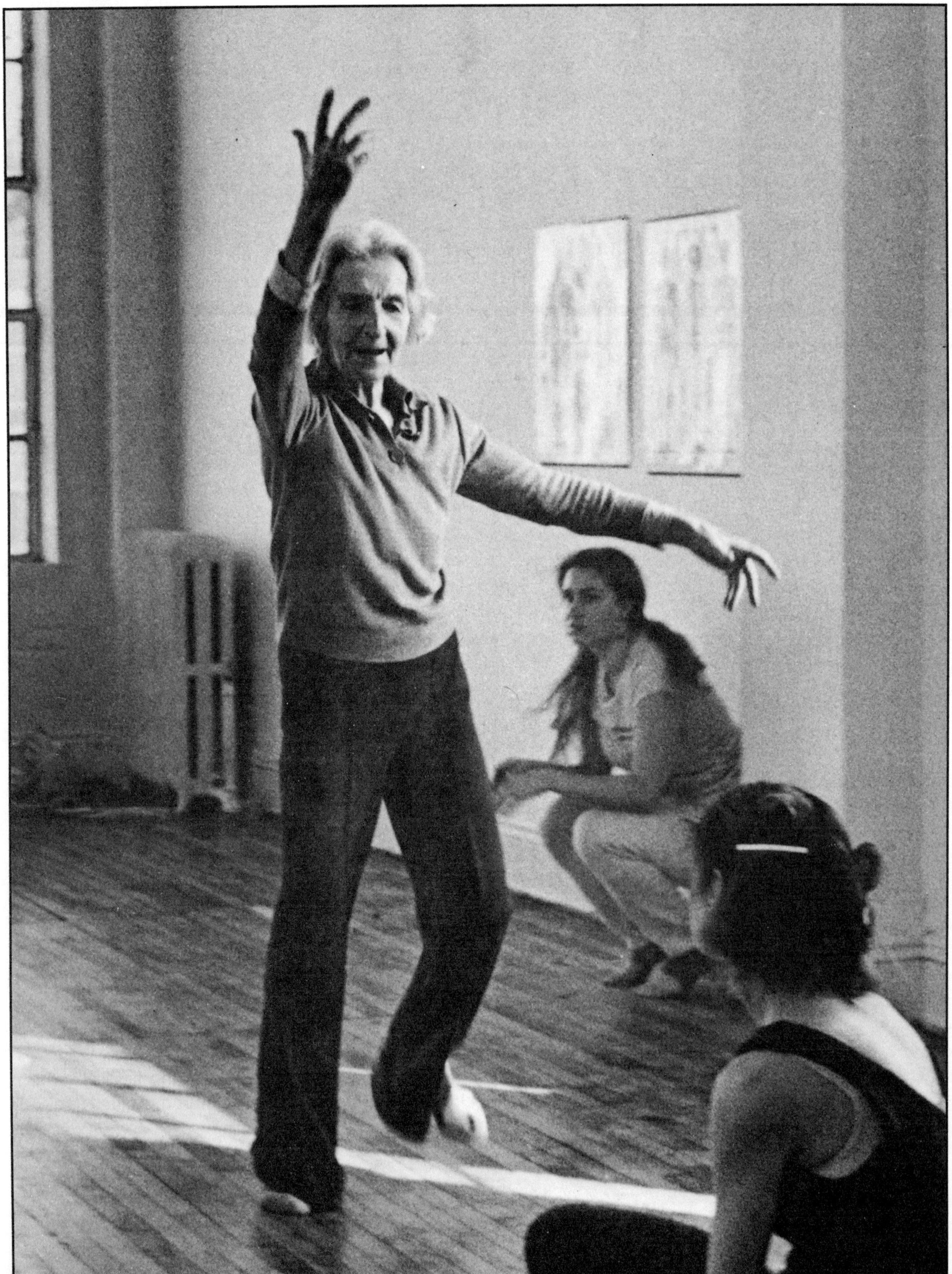

PHOTO COURTESY OF DEBORAH DAY

Movement can make a significant and important contribution both to the older adult and society as a whole.

- There are special physical, psychological and social needs such ass depression and isolation that an effective dance program can serve.

- The myths of aging need to be reexamined.

- There is a need for research dissemination on the impact of dance and the older adult population.

Conference Presentors

Sheila E. Barnett: M.A., Director-Jamaica School of Dance, Cultural Training Centre; Written, choreographed and presented T.V. programs for skills development for dance teachers and cultural dynamics in education; Planned and organized first Caribbean Dance Seminar held in Jamaica, sponsored by O.A.S.; Visiting Artist to Britain, for lecture tour including workshops, master classes and seminars funded by Commonwealth foundation; Formerly principal dancer for the National Dance Theatre Company of Jamaica; Choreographer-National Dance Theatre Company of Jamaica.

Dianne A.R. Bartley: Ph.D., Assistant Professor in Exercise Physiology with an emphasis in Nutrition; Taught at the University of Maryland for 12 years; Presently in the Department of Physical Education and Recreation at Howard University.

Monica Belthran: M.A., ADTR, Therapist and Consultant; Dance Movement Therapist for past 7 years; Used expressive therapy with Geriatrics and Medical Rehabilitative population in in/out patient settings; Developed dance movement program for 250 bed nursing home in Baltimore, Maryland and later extended work to include senior citizens; Presently, Coordinator of a Psychological-Social Program for traumatically injured adults at Baltimore Rehabilitative Center for Living; Clinical Supervisor for the Dance Movement Therapy Program at Goucher College; Program Director for metropolitan area American Dance Therapy Association.

Sherrill Berryman-Miller: Ph.D., Conference Coordinator; Assistant Professor of Dance, Department of Physical Education, Howard University; Responsible for presenting professional dance companies at Howard University and providing expertise in scholarly research on dance in the areas of history, humanities, and gerontology.

Lydia Bragger: Chairperson of the National Grey Panthers Media Watch; challenged and changed much of the age stereotyping prevalent in the media through the production of radio and television programs, appearances on David Suskind and other T.V. shows, and articles on aging.

Linda Eanello: M.A., Teacher at The Sacred Heart School; New York State Chair for the National Dance Association-Alliance of Health, Physical Education, Recreation and Dance.

Beth S. Eubanks: M.A., Member of the faculty in the Department of Physical Education at Howard University for past 11 years; Presently completing Ph.D. in Therapeutic Recreation and Gerontology at the University of Maryland, College Park.

Milton Feher: Creator of Effortless Motion Therapy, and director of the Milton Feher School of Dance and Relaxation; graduated from the Neighborhood Playhouse School of Theater in 1934. In curing arthritis of his knee, devised a system of relaxing and strengthening the entire body.

Michael L. Freedman: M.D., Professor and Director of the Division of Geriatric Medicine at N.Y.U. Medical Center, and Co-Director of CARE (Center for Care of the Aged - Research and Education); Editorial Board Member for the Journal of Nutrition for the Elderly; Founding member, American Federation for Aging Research.

Margie Hanson: Ph.D., Vice President of the American Alliance of Health, Recreation, Physical Education and Dance; Elementary Education Consultant since 1965; Executive Director of the National Dance Association since 1971.

Leah Harpaz: M.A., Dance Therapist; Teacher of Movement for Older Adults at 92nd Street Y; Co-Author, Therapeutic Dance/Movement, Co-Producer of two records; Adjunct lecturer at Adelphi University and C.U.N.Y.; conducts workshops throughout the United States and Israel.

Estelle Harriton: Teacher of International Folk Dancing; studied at the Neighborhood Playhouse; former member of the Children's Theater of the WPA Dance Project; legal secretary; returned with enthusiasm in her 70's to teach folk dance to her contemporaries.

Bernadette Hecox: B.S., M.A., Associate Professor in Clinical Physical Therapy at Columbia University; Teacher of Anatomy and Movement Analysis at The Julliard School; Private dance studio director, physical therapist, lecturer, book consultant, T.V. personality.

Jocelyn B. Helm: M.A., Certified in Movement Rehabilitation; Dance Therapist, Director of the Princeton Senior Resource Center; President, Gerontological Society of New Jersey, member of Sigma Phi Omega (honorary gerontological society), New Jersey delegate to the National Council on Aging.

Eileen Jones: M.A., Teacher, Laban Movement Analysis, Trained by Betty Meridith-Jones; Instructor at the Jung Foundation, The Gestalt Institute, Columbia University, and The New School for Social Research; Teacher of Movement for Older Adults at Riverside Church and St. Patrick's Cathedral.

Shabaka Jones-El: Graduate of University of Massachusetts; Learned Yang style of the art of Tai Chi Chuan from Robert Cheng, Chicago, Illinois; 16 year practitioner in the art of Tai Chi; Taught at Barney Senior Center, Judiciary House and Friendship Terrace Apts. for the Elderly, Roosevelt for Senior Citizens; Presently teaching at Washington Senior Wellness Center, St. Mary's Court, Multi-Arts Program, and N.Y. Presbyterian Church.

Jack Kallish: Teacher of Dance for Older Adults at Henry Street Playhouse, Educational Alliance, United Jewish Council; Social Worker and Recreation Leader at Senior Centers, Department of Aging, and CARING.

Liz Lerman: M.A., Artistic Director of The Dance Exchange, Washington, D.C.; Choreographer and founder of the troupe "Dancers for the Third Age"; Author of Teaching Dance to Senior Citizens (1984). Her approach blends theater (mime, jazz, voice) with dance.

Marcia b. Leventhal: Ph.D., A.D.T.R.-C.M.A.; Associate Professor, Department of Dance and Dance Education, New York University, and Director of Graduate Dance Therapy Program at NYU and abroad in Stockholm, Sweden; Editor, "Movement and Growth: Dance Therapy for the Special Child" Chair of Special Services, Dance Therapy Committee, N.D.A.

Jed A. Levine: M.A., CPTR; Supervisor of the Day Treatment at the International Center for the Disabled in New York. Specialist in therapeutic recreation, reality orientation, and drama therapy for older adults. Lecturer and workshop leader at colleges and universities in the U.S.

Erna Caplow Lindner: M.S., ACSE, Professor at Nassau Community College and Adelphi University; dance Therapy Consultant and Trainer for geriatric, rehabilitative, educational, and residential care institutions. Co-Author, Therapeutic Dance/Movement, and co-producer of two records.

Andrew AA. Monjan: M.P.H., Ph.D., Chief Neurobiology and Immunology Programs, Neuroscience of Aging Branch, National Institute on Aging; Expert-Epidemiology, Extramural Programs of the Cerebellum and LCM Virus Cerebullar Disease in Neonates; Cited in American Men and Women in Science and Who's Who in Frontier Science and Technology; Member of American Association for the Advancement of Science and Society for Neuroscience.

Lot Bates Page: M.D., Special Assistant to the Director, National Institute on Aging, NIH; Professor of Medicine, Tufts University, School of Medicine; Professional Publications' "Salt and Drinking Water", "Dietary Sodium and Blood Pressure: Evidence from Human Studies", "The Hazards of Hypertension and the Determinants of Blood Pressure in Populations", "Can Hypertension by Prevented".

Robert Perez: Ph.D., Exercise Physiologist and Assistant Professor at Adelphi University; Adjunct Lecturer at Brooklyn College. Researcher on sports-medicine; developed guidelines for adult fitness programs for the institutionalized elderly and for master athletes.

Jacquelin Portis: M.Ed, RMT-BC, Board-Certified Registered Music Therapist in the field for 10 years; Worked as a music therapist, private music therapy consultant, workshop leader and served as Music Therapy Clinical Training Director, St. Elizabeth's Hospital, Division of Child and Adolescent Services; Responsible for training and supervision of music therapy interns; Member of National Association for Music Therapy; Worked extensively with geriatric population; Presently Educational-vocational Specialist with Residential Adolescent Substance Abuse Treatment Program in Washington, D.C.

Susan L. Sandel: Ph.D., ADTR, Administrator, New Haven Convalescent Center; Co-Director, Creative Psycho-Therapy Center; Faculty, University of New Haven and Antioch-New England Graduate School. Her work with nursing home residents is portrayed in ADTA's film "Dance Therapy: The Power Of Movement".

Judith G. Schwartz: M.A., Conference Chairperson; Associate Professor of Dance and Dance Education at New York University; Specialist in Dance for Children and Older Adults; Director and Founder of Kaleidescope Dancers; U.S. Representative, Dance and The Child International; Co-Chair, N.D.A. Children's Task Force on Dance.

Allen Sher: Ed.D., Organizer of Vermont Governor's Council on Physical Fitness; Workshop leader for Folk Dancing and Senior Citizens; Member of Ed Larkin Contra Dancers - a group that demonstrates contra dances, quadrilles, and round dances of Vermont and New England.

Delfa Vaznaugh: Works extensively in hospital and institutional settings to improve the quality of care through movement; Developed workshops for hospital personnel to emphasize the need to renew day-to-day patterns of movement; Lectured in Canada, Brazil, and the United States; Held workshops with Catholic University, National Hispanic Council on Aging, Association of Occupational Therapists of Quebec, the Universite of Montreal, and West Texas Council on the Aging.

Dale Walkonen: M.A., Conference Coordinator; Free lance Writer, Mime, Newscaster and Artistic Director for "The One Show", Manhattan Cable Television.